YOU'RE MISSING

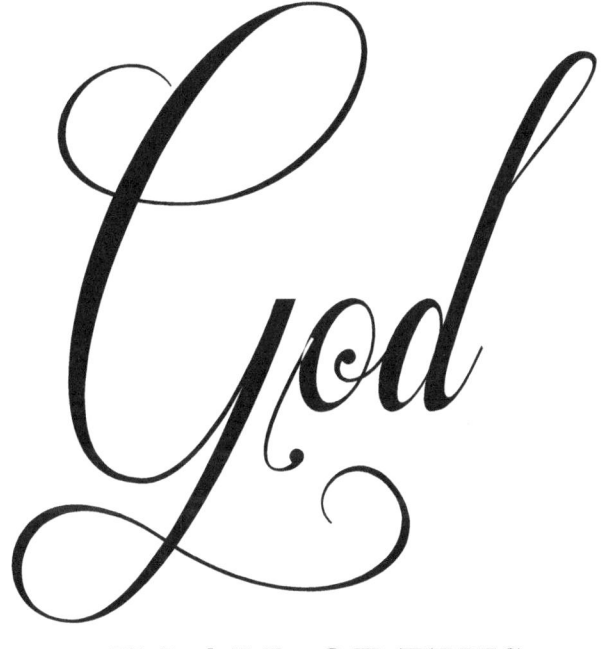

IN ALL OF THIS

THE STORY THAT HAD TO BE TOLD

LYDIA M. LEWIS

PUBLISHED BY FIDELI PUBLISHING INC.

© Copyright 2013 Lydia Lewis

All Rights Reserved.

No part of this book may be reproduced, stored in a retrieval system, or transmitted by any means, electronic, mechanical, photocopying, recording, or otherwise, without written permission from the author.

ISBN: 978-1-60414-735-3

Table of Contents

Acknowledgements .... *v*
Introduction .... *vii*

The Story Begins 1
Lee (Like His Name) a Lion 5
Angels 9
Another Tragedy 11
The Relationship 18
Prayer Request 22
The Love Letter 24
"Come Clean' 30
Our Weekend 32
Trouble in Paradise 35
Take a Chance 37
Movie Scene 45
The Wait 50
The Awakening 56
Wedding Plans 59
The Operating Room Again 61
Rehab Again 63
Obama For My Man 69
Visitors From the Big Apple 71
Rehab? 74

I Messed Up!	78
Time to Move	81
Is This a Problem?	83
Reality Check	85
When We Get Married	89
Prosthesis/Lawyer	90
"Nobody Knows"	91
Great Love	93
Still Waiting	96
"Lord, Please Give Ernie a Break"	105
Home for Thanksgiving	108
One More Time	111
The End?	120
Dedication	123

Acknowledgements

Heartfelt thanks to those who never stopped praying, never stopped calling, never stopped sending cards, and never stopped visiting during my husband's lengthy illness. We were truly blessed to have you in our lives. I am not going to list names. You know, we know and more important, God knows who your are. For those who dispensed with church jargon and spiritually correct remarks passed down through the years but simply held my hand or gave me a hug and said, "Lydia, Sis Lewis, or my sister, I am praying for you." I thank you, that was what I needed more than anything.

Introduction

I always enjoyed writing. When I was in Junior High, I joined a creative writing club and even had a few of my writings and poems published in our school newsletter. So, I thought it was not strange when I was encouraged by my three cousins, Edna, Roger and Calvin who said, "You have to write the story."

These promptings vividly brought back to me in September 2010 as Reverend Lewis was being rushed to the OR as I was running beside him by his stretcher he looked up and said, "You have to tell the story."

I replied, "I can't tell it like you."

He just repeated, "You have to tell the story."

God is good. He survived that surgery and we were blessed with two more years, and two more months and six more days together. When he told the story, some people even cried, some felt hopeful and some just enjoyed the enchantment of it. They too said, "You need to write a book about it. So here I am trying to tell the story to the very best of my ability.

About a year and a half into Ernest's hospitalizations, our constant prayer was that the Lord would restore him to the health he enjoyed before the surgery. With one set back after another, and the realization that it may not be part of God's plan Ernest shared with me, "If I ever get a chance to preach another sermon, I would title it 'You're Missing God In All Of This.'" He said, "We've gone through more in the few years we've been together than couples married 20, 30, 40, 50, 60 years. They just don't have a clue!" He never got a chance to preach that sermon, but he lived it by witnessing to the hand of God, "In All Of This."

The Story Begins

In April of 2001, I became employed part time, at Kennedy Health System as a registered nurse, in their outpatient Dialysis Unit. I looked forward to being employed so close to home, because. I no longer had to commute from New Jersey to Philadelphia ,which I had endured since October of 1987.

Previously I was employed at the Hospital of University of Pennsylvania acute dialysis unit until it was sold. I worked at HUP as it is frequently called for 24 years and I thought I would retire from there. As we say in nursing, "We plan, God laughs." After about six months, a full time position became available at Kennedy and I applied and I was hired full time.

Being the "low nurse on the staffing ladder," I was often the one asked to work at another Kennedy outpatient unit when they were short staffed. I really didn't mind because it actually was a refreshing change. The staff there was friendly, kind and supportive. The patients, well patients are basically the same wherever you work.

That's where I first met Ernest W. Lewis the 1st. He was one of several patients I cared for. He was dialyzed Monday, Wednesday, and Friday, first shift. I remembered him as we identified patients as a "walkie-talkie." He was self-sufficient and friendly.

On my many "floats" from my unit in Washington Township to Stratford, he gave me a copy of his book *How to Handle Stress* and a few CDs. He confessed several years later that he was flirting with me, but I had no clue. I thought he was just being friendly. More importantly I recognized him from the beginning as being a real "people person."

Ernest later admitted that because I didn't respond to his advances, he asked another nurse that worked, Jasmine, at the Stratford dialysis center, about me. She told him, "Leave her alone she's married."

Jasmine invited him to visit Christ Care Unit Missionary Baptist Church, a.k.a. C.C.U., where Rev. Dr. Robert F. Hargrove Sr., is the Pastor and Founder. He accepted the invitation and saw for himself that I was married. My husband, Leon, and our three children all were members. Ernest joined C.C.U. and became one of the associate ministers.

Ernest's health declined and he became a victim of what we in nursing call the "chop shop." First, he had one toe amputated, then another, and then a foot and his leg. In Ernest's case, his amputation was below the knee. Then the same scenario repeated itself on the other leg. Again, first the toes, then the foot and then the leg. Fortunately again it was below the knee.

Below the knee made it possible for him to be fitted for a prosthesis. He had his personalized, one with a picture of his mom, Ernestine, and the other with his family tree.

Even with the bilateral amputations, he was determined to maintain his independence. No pity party for him! He had his own apartment, took care of his personal needs, cooked and shopped. He had a motorized wheelchair and could be seen cruising up and down Sicklerville Road. He used Access Link and New Jersey Transit to go shopping, to the mall, and to take care of business.

His apartment was in the church's senior housing which was located right behind the church. He was also faithful in attending services. If the truth were to be told, he was at more services than those in much better health and with mobility. He came out in the summer heat and winter cold. He was there not just on Sundays. Occasionally, he joined the prayer warriors on Monday nights, attended Wednesday Bible study, Friday evening services, revivals, home going services and when possible visited other churches when we were invited.

He truly loved the Lord. Ernest praised the Lord and committed himself to serve the Lord with all his heart, mind and soul. He later told me that when the Lord called him in the ministry in 1986, the Lord told him, "I have use of your life and your testimony."

His first sermon on June15 1986 was "Living to live again." He truly sought to live for Christ. On his business card he had "I just want to do God's will."

His love for God and people allowed him to witness very comfortably to individuals of all walks of life regardless of race, gender or age. He was very "down to earth" and that allowed him to plant a seed. The scripture that he shared the most was Ecclesiastes 3: 1-13. ([1]To everything *there is* a season, A time for every purpose under heaven.)

This was the same scripture my sixth grade graduating class memorized and recited at our commencement.

He used Compact Discs as his icebreaker. He was very computer savvy and burned more CD›s than even he ever knew. Only the Lord knows how many. Old hymns, contemporary gospel, some jazz and R&B too. Sorry to shock some of you super saints, but he loved music. His record collection was overwhelming. He must have had about a hundred albums. When it came to music he could hang with the best, knowing artists and dates. To him music had no color.

Lee (Like His Name) a Lion

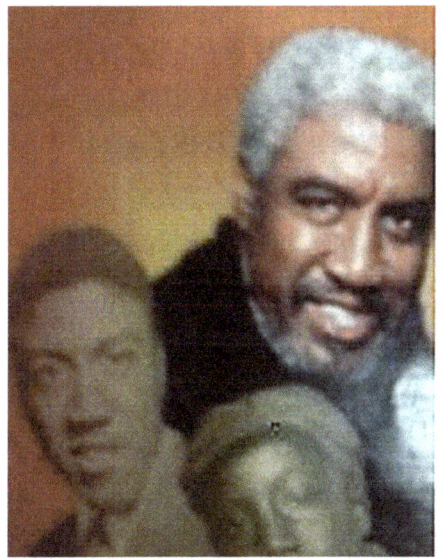

My first husband, Leon B. Howard Sr. of 35 years, one month and 29 days died after a very brief illness.

Our courtship began when I was in college. He loved to write poetry and he wrote this poem to me when I was at Hampton.

Lydia baby my beautiful dove
A gift to me from heaven above
You're nice and loving, this I know
My love for you I try to show
Your charm and grace is beyond compare
Not only here but everywhere
I love you baby and I can see
That you're the girl that's meant for me
I'm trying to do the best I can
To make you proud of the average man
I know there's more that could be done
Like entertainment, amusement and fun
These things we think of but seldom speak
Shall come to pass you will see
So love me baby like I love you
Soon college lessons you won't have to do
In conclusion my beautiful dove
I send my love, kisses and hugs

He fell at home on April 11, 2005, was admitted to the hospital in April for mental status changes and pneumonia. On the 21st, he was transferred to Rehab then readmitted to the hospital because of electrolyte imbalances. Then he went back to Rehab on the 27th and then finally stabilized and was discharged home on the 12th of May. Then he fell again on the 28th of May and was taken to the ER diagnosed with a subdural hematoma and immediately transferred to Thomas Jefferson Hospital in Philadelphia for surgery.

Even though the surgery was needed right away, it was delayed because of his clotting factors. His surgery was performed on June 1st, and according to the surgeons all went well.

He coded the 3rd of June and died. I thank God for Nylin Tennessee who came as soon as I called her. She drove my family to the hospital in the rain. She did not like driving in the rain, but out of love she did it for me and my family. Sis. Paula Hargrove also came as soon as she found out and supported me in such a loving manner and in so many ways.

Even to this day, Rev. Bright, my former pastor, reflects on the kindness he witnessed by our first lady during my time of sorrow. So, as you can imagine, his death was a tremendous shock. Lee, as I affectionately called him, was the father of our three children: Leon Bernard Howard Jr., Leona Brenda Howard and Lynette Belinda Howard.

Lee loved the Lord and was a staunch defender of God's written word. He was a bold and outspoken soldier for the Lord. Everyone who knew him recognized that. One of the sisters took me to the side after a church meeting and said, "Bro. Howard is just saying what so many others are thinking, but just don't have the 'guts' to spit it out." He often challenged those who did not present God's Word in its proper context. He spent hours studying the Bible.

He had such a passion for the word of God that he held a summer Bible class for children on our patio when we lived in Philadelphia. He felt strongly that all Christians had a call to minister. Not necessarily from a pulpit but from wherever they were. It became so popular that one Jehovah Witness attended on occasion. I assisted him by serving homemade brownies and lemonade.

He loved his family. From the beginning of our relationship he made it clear how much he wanted children. He enjoyed taking care of them, cooking "big breakfasts" for them, playing games with them, being there for their activities, attending back to school nights, etc. He enjoyed writing poetry especially of family and life in general.

He positioned himself as our protector and defender. His sudden death drove me into a depression and life seemed too much to bear. I sought God and psychiatric counseling. Some people speak so negatively of psychiatric intervention, but when you have a toothache, you pray and go to the dentist. So when you know your mind is disturbed and consider hurting yourself or someone else, you should pray and get help. A good psychiatrist or psychoanalyst will allow you to talk, will lead you to the point where you recognize the problem and see a solution.

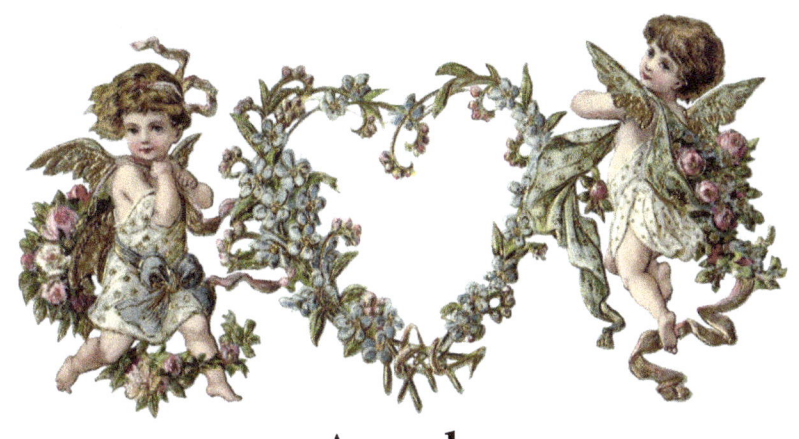

Angels

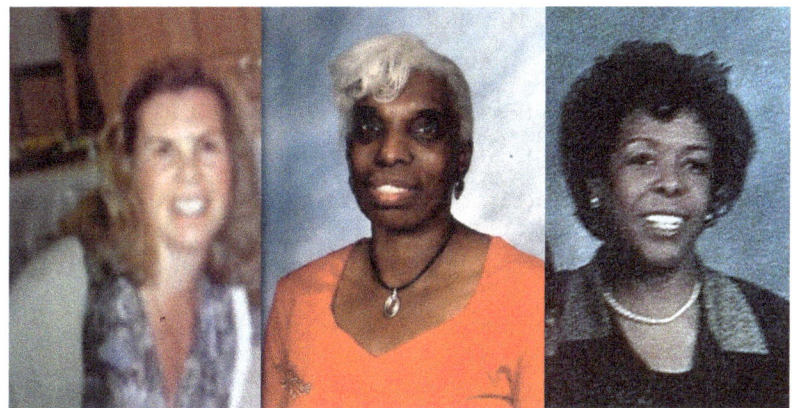

I continued to work at Kennedy after Lee passed away. Upon my arrival to the unit at 4:30 a.m., one of my initial tasks was to check the patient census to see if any of our patients had been admitted. Each time I saw Rev. Lewis's name, I either went to visit him or sent him a card. He appreciated the "book cards" especially and asked me to pick up some for him to send to the sick and bereaved.

I gladly did and also gave him the name and number of the Christian bookstore that I frequented in Glassboro.

After several visits to him in the hospital, he informed me that I had become one of his "angels." He announced, "And now, I have three."

Jasmine F., RN, was another nurse who often took care of him in dialysis when he was admitted. He appreciated the excellent care she gave him and enjoyed so much their conversations and Christian fellowship.

Also, Judi Dowell called him every Monday to check on him after his first dialysis treatment of the week. Judi has shown her faithfulness in all that the Lord assigns her to do. She gave Ernest two angels while he was admitted to the hospital, "An angel from an angel," he would say. (They now have a home in our office on the top shelf of one of our bookcases.) And lastly, me, for checking on him when he was admitted. He jokingly said, "You always find me."

Another Tragedy

After prayer with the Prayer Warriors on Monday, July 22 2007, I returned home and saw that I had missed a call from my younger daughter, Lynette. She had left a message that she was in a lot of pain and was going to the emergency room. I said to myself, *I'll wait a bit and call her to see what's going on.*

I dozed off only to be awakened by a phone call from Atlantic City Hospital. They asked what relation I was to Lynette. Being awakened out of a deep sleep, I answered, "Her sister." I then quickly corrected myself and said, "No, I'm her mother."

The lady said, "She's here at Atlantic City Hospital. Please come and bring someone with you."

When she said that, I felt like my heart was about to

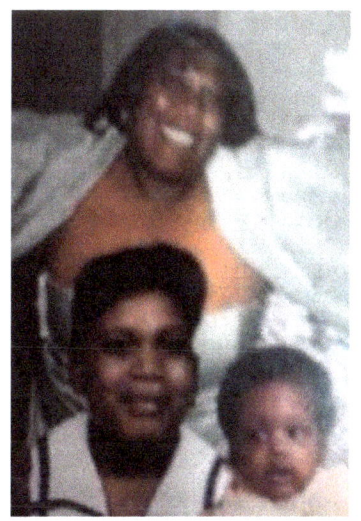

explode out of my chest. I said, "Where is Atlantic City Hospital?"

She said, "It's right across from Caesars." Then she repeated, "Bring someone with you."

Right then and there I felt my legs go limp. I called my daughter, Leona, and then my daughter in-love, Cheryl, and told them about the phone call. Cheryl rushed over and made the decision that the men should stay behind. That would be Leon, my son, Darnell, Leona's husband, Lamont and Kenny Wayne, my grandsons. They were instructed to pray and we would call them as soon as we found out what was going on.

Honestly, it seemed like Cheryl drove and got us there in 15 minutes versus the usual 30 to 45 minutes it takes. When we arrived, a doctor and nurse took us in a room and the worst fear a mother could have was realized. Lynette was dead.

We all, just like with my husband Lee, couldn't believe it. We screamed. We cried. We were hysterical. We finally calmed down and they took us in to see her. She had the most beautiful smile that I had ever seen. She looked so at peace. Cheryl sent up a prayer in that room that touched everyone present.

The doctor said Lynette had a pulmonary embolus. We found out later that she called 911, then called me, and then took the elevator down to the 1st floor. Her apartment was on the 16th. She went outside and collapsed in the street, 911 came and rushed her to the hospital. She coded, but they could not save her.

She was fine the day before. She rushed in to C.C.U. after working, she was a waitress at the Tropicana. She took the bus because her car was in the shop, and exclaimed as she entered the church, "I made it!"

After the 8 o clock service, she took my car, ran some errands and got some sleep at my house. That evening, I drove her back to Avandale Park 'n Ride to return to Atlantic City. She had to work. The next morning, I called her and thanked her for putting gas in my car, She said, "No problem." I told her I would talk to her later in the week and that I loved her and I hung up.

Lynette was a beautiful, vivacious young lady. She was hard working and ambitious. She was an avid movie "goer" and had dreamed of becoming a movie critic. She had already applied to several schools and had started to save money for an apartment she saw online in North Carolina.

God knows I had a real hard time with her death. I screamed out to God, "You took my only brother (1972), my parents (1990), my only sister (1999) my husband, and now my youngest daughter! Who's next?" I was so devastated by her death that I couldn't write her obituary. I used her personal statement for schools to which she applied.

Lydia M. Lewis

Obituary

Personal Statement
Written by Lynette B. Howard

"I was born by the river, in a little tent, and just like the river, I've been running ever since. It's been a long time coming, and I know a change will come." Sam Cooke wrote these lyrics in 1964, and I don't think any other song can describe my life better.

I was born in September of 1979 by the Delaware River in Philadelphia, PA. At the age of 8, my family moved to New Jersey. After graduation from high school is where I began my race...."and been running ever since".

Being born the youngest of 3 children, I was able to look to my older siblings for guidance, and was always encouraged to follow my heart and dream big. Silly of me, I chose the 'Show me the money" sate of mind. For this reason, my heart was not into college in 1997. So, I decided to take time off to "find myself". I wanted to know exactly what I want to do with the rest of my life. This journey stretched across 5 states and lasted for 10 years. All this time, and what do I get, "another day older and deeper in debt."

In February of 2005, I returned to New Jersey from Louisiana and decided not to travel for a while. I spent time meditating and soul searching to figure out what makes me happiest, because I was destined to complete my education. In June of that same year, my father passed away from an in-house infection he caught while recovering from brain surgery.

My father had a love of films. The first video I owned was given to me as a Christmas present from him. Now "Beauty & and the Beast" is the first of over 400 videos I own in my collection, and it is still one of my favorites.

(I think I have found my passion in life.)

My father introduced me to Dorothy Dandridge before Halle Berry introduced her to the world. I would watch AMC and TCM and we would chat about the old classics. He would tell me about films he saw as a child and his favorite actors/actresses. In his latter years, he couldn't sit still in a theater. So, I would go to the cinemas and come back and tell him about them.

There is not a day that goes by that I don't miss him. I still tell him about the movies though. Instead of telling him face to face, I write them down, revise them, and turn them into reviews. I post them on my webpage: **www.myspace.com/acsafire**

I dream of being a film critic. It took me 10 years to find what I was passionate about, and now I can't imagine wanting to do anything else.

Isaiah 40:31 But they that wait upon the Lord shall renew their strength; they shall mount up with wings as eagles; they shall run, and not be weary; and they shall walk, and not faint."

I was confident her soul was secure and that she was with her daddy in heaven. She wrote this poem a month before she died. We included it in her home going service.

I Remember

He left us so quick
Without a blink of warning,
His body was tired,
And his soul was ready for departing.

As the time passed
And tears have been shed,
My mind started to wander,
And here is where it led.

Being awoken each morning
With the bellow in his tones.
As he walked me to school
We sang of the fire shut up in our bones.

At Dinnertime, our tummies
Were filled quite nice.
With entrees so tasty,
Like his infamous Spanish Rice.

Emeril can't spice up
And Rachael Ray can't quicken
The recipes of delights
That came out of our kitchen.

We moved out of Philly
With the help of his VA,
With dreams of a better future
For his children one day.

We went to see the 76ers attempt to win,
And the Harlem Globetrotters play.
Watching the Eagles on the tube.
Hoping they would win the Superbowl one day.

It has been 2 years since your exit.
And when I reflect back.
These are a sample of the memories
I pull out of my sack.

Even though you are no longer with us,
I just wanted to say.
I'll remember you always,
And Happy Father's Day!

Lydia M. Lewis

"I was blessed when she wrote this Essay about me.

Lynette Howard
Essay
"What African-American person has been an inspiration to you and why?"

What African-American person has been an inspiration to you and why?

  The African-American person that has had the biggest influence on my life, would be no one other than my mother. My mother, Lydia Mae McMillan Howard, is one of the smartest, bravest, strongest people in the world. Maybe I am just being biased because she is my mother, but please allow me to explain.

  My mother was born the daughter of Ruby and Augusta McMillan. She is the eldest of three children. Her mother, Ruby, had a disease called epilepsy. After seeing what her mother went through with this disease, she decided that she wanted to go to school to become a doctor and cure the illness.

  She grew up in a time in which it was a crime for a black woman to be well educated. Blacks were subject to the worst of everything. They had the worst neighborhoods, the worst schools, the worst foods. However they made do with what they had..

  After graduating from high school, Lydia Mae went off to college at Hampton University, but at the time it was known at Hampton Institute. Here is where she obtained her Bachelor's in Science degree.

  Since then, my mother has gotten married and had 3 children. She made sure that her children had clothes on their back, roof over their heads, and food in their mouths. She moved us out of the city and into the suburbs. We had the advantage of living in a nice neighborhood with good schools. My mother has remained at the same job for over 20 years, showing us children that stability in the workplace is possible. All three children graduated from high school and went on for advancements in education.

  My mother made it through the murder of her young brother, the death of her parents, and the death of her younger sister. Her husband and children are the only immediate family she has left, and she shows us all how much we mean to her everyday.

  In conclusion, I could have chosen Martin Luther King or Malcolm X. You know, someone a little more well known, but I decided to choose someone who is known well by me. My mother is a well-educated black female. She is strong and determined. She let all the things that occurred in her life make her stronger instead of weakening her spirit, characteristics that I hope to withhold within myself. My mother is my life, because she gave me life.

  I know that she will not be here forever, and I don't know when she will leave my life. I do know, however, that while she is here I will praise her. I will be thankful for all she has done. Why wait until she is gone to show her my love and appreciation.

She gave me my flowers while I could smell them."

About a week after Lynette's service, one of my co-worker's daughter died. She was about 12 years old and had required 24 hour nursing care with technical support all her life. I attended the service and my co-workers were surprised to see me. As Rick Warrren said in his book *The Purpose Driven Life* "It's not about me." The preacher said something that day that truly spoke to my grief "When a parent loses a child, there is a hole that will always remain in their heart". I signed a release for Lynette's organs to be donated. Since then I have been comforted in knowing that her skin has helped burn victims and her bones for knee transplants.

The Relationship

My life continued. God was merciful and slow to anger. I asked His forgiveness for my outburst.

"The Lord giveth and the Lord taketh, blessed be the name of the Lord." — Job 1:21

I still worked at Kennedy, and was looking forward to retiring in a few years. I was done taking seminary classes. Actually, Rev. Lewis and I attended a few together and I remained active *in* the various ministries to which I belonged and community outreach programs.

In the spring of 2010, I saw the movie "The book of Eli" starring Denzel Washington. I enjoyed it so much that I decided to purchase a DVD and give it to Rev. Lewis for his birthday.

Our acquaintanceship had grown. It would be a smile and a handshake as I passed him, and when I went up for offering, more smiles and more smiles. Despite my efforts, the DVD wasn't available yet. So, on June 2nd, two days before his birthday, after Bible Study I gave him a birthday card with an IOU that said, "IOU 'The book of ELI DVD when it comes out." When it did become available, I purchased it and gave it to him.

Our acquaintanceship continued, and one Sunday he approached me and said, "You didn't shake my hand today when you went around for offering."

I apologized, smiled and said, "It won't happen again."

One Wednesday evening after Bible study, I was in the copy room. He was wheeling by, and he saw me and came in to tell me again how much he appreciated my acts of kindness during his many hospitalizations. He invited me to his apartment to see how he had displayed the various cards and gifts I had given him.

I simply smiled and said to myself, *I know this preacher is not inviting me to his apartment. What will the residents at C.C.U. Senior Housing think?*

He approached me a week later and apologized, saying, "I hope I didn't offend you; but you know you have to come and watch the movie with me." I accepted his invitation and we were tentatively trying to set a date.

Before we found a time good for the both of us, he asked me to meet him at St. James, a neighboring church. They were having a weekend gospel fest, an outdoor service that Saturday and a Sunday afternoon service. I told him I had to work that Saturday, but I could meet him there after work. I went home excited about the prospect of spending the afternoon with him away from C.C.U.

Well, that Saturday at work it was so busy and so hectic that at 2:30 p.m. when I should have been done, being in charge, I had some things I really had to finish up. I called him and apologized, and told him how crazy it was at work that day. I said I didn't think I'd be good company for anyone by the time I got off. He sounded disappointed, but said OK.

We saw each other at church the next day, and again I apologized. He jokingly said, "You 'owe me.' You stood me up yesterday, so you can't deny me. Let's go to the diner and get a bite to eat and then go to their afternoon service."

Without hesitation, I said, "Yes, that would be nice."

That was on June 27, 2010. That day I will remember until I'm old and drooling in my oatmeal. We sat in his booth, the last one on the left as you enter the diner. It was the largest space in that part of the diner and it made it easier for him to transfer from his wheelchair to the booth.

I ordered a salad, not knowing how his funds were. We were at the end of the month. He ordered a big, hearty meal. He was a real meat and potato man, with cheesecake for dessert.

We literally sat there for hours. It was a quiet Sunday afternoon so we weren't made to feel like we were monopolizing a table. We laughed, talked and talked, and laughed some more. We finally abandoned the idea of going to the afternoon service. The love bug flew in and bit both of us.

When he told the story, he said I proposed to him. Honestly I don't remember that, I can't imagine myself doing that, but I could have, because I felt on that day that God had placed someone in my life to love and be committed to forever and ever. When we finally left the diner, it was getting dark.

Prayer Request

It was January 24, 2010, I can't remember if it was at a church setting or a prayer group, but we were instructed to write down two things that we were struggling with and pray for God's intervention. We were told to place it in our Bibles and to keep praying and wait on the Lord's answer. I wrote loneliness and poor self-esteem and placed it in my new Bible given to me by the Dance Ministry.

Rose Bridget Brady was an Irish American senior citizen that I adopted while working at HUP. I passed her house daily as I walked to work after parking my car in that area. She would give me snacks in the morning and I would stop by after work for a few minutes and chat and pray with her. She was single, never married, and she always said she saw "their faults too soon." She never had any children and she was lonely. She told me on several occasions, "Lydia, loneliness is the worst disease there is." I had learned, like millions all over the world, that she was right.

Loneliness is something the church doesn't even address. When public prayer requests are solicited, they are for the sick, bereaved, marriages, youth, finances, and seniors, but never as a young sister once dared to say at a Wednesday night Bible class, the lonely hearted. I guess it is so much easier to ignore or pretend that that group doesn't exist.

Bonnie Mills, Mae Billingsley and I attended a weekend retreat sponsored by Min. Pam Carter. We were roommates. During one of our private girlie sessions in our room, I shared some of the advances from men since my husband Leon had died. Bonnie said, "Lydia you need a man spiritually more mature than you, not someone you have to bring up to your level."

That conversation came vividly to mind when my relationship with Ernest evolved. Was he the one Bonnie spoke of? Was he the answer to that first part of my prayer, loneliness?

The Love Letter

If there was any doubt that Ernest loved me, he dismissed it with this letter.

> June 29, 2010, 6:27am

Dearest Lydia,

 I do hope and pray that this letter finds you in the blessed precious care of our Lord and Savior Jesus Christ. I have been so blessed over these past few days, even months, at just what God has done in our lives. It is so amazing how God has moved in your life, with regards towards your feelings for me!

 I am not much on letter writing, but there was something that came to my mind this morning and I wanted you to know just what it was. I am a big romantic person, as you have said you are also, so a few songs were floating around in my head while thinking about "**YOU**"

There was this song called "*I Do Love you,*" by **Billy Steward**. Some of the words went like this, "I do love you, with all my heart, yes I do, now," and that's the way I feel about you, NOW! Another song that was in my heart is, "***When We Get Married,***" by **Larry Graham &Grand Central Station**, with these words"

> "When we get married,
> we'll have a big celebration,
> Send invitations to all our friends'
> and relations.
> We'll have a ball dancing and all
> when we get married!"

Couldn't remember all the words but I do hope that you seeing where I am going. I've come this far and I am not turning back. I'm in this for the long haul. I truly believe in my heart that God Himself has ordained this marriage! I have waited just for "***YOU***" we belong together. ***AMEN!***

Thanks from the bottom of my heart for what has transpired so far, and I am eagerly looking forward to the next hour and the next day, and the next week, and the next month and the years to come! There is no doubt in my heart at this point that I have fallen in "**LOVE**" with "**YOU.**"

Let's see just where God is taking us. I do believe in my heart there is a joyful life ahead for us. Let's take each other's hand and press toward the mark of the high calling in Christ Jesus!

We deserve to have life and have it more abundantly. Like you said, life is too short, and living it alone is not too pleasing. If you will have me, I ain't gonna go nowhere! Just a few words from my heart to your heart.

Precious Care, Precious Prayer,
Precious Love

Always in Christ Jesus, Ernest

We had found love and it was the love we always wanted.

Again, I fell on my knees thanking God for sending me a Man of God who loved the Lord with all of his heart, mind and soul and had entrusted his heart and feelings to me. Not only was I blessed, Matthew 5:45 reminds us that God allows the rain to fall on the just as well as the unjust, but I felt like Mary highly favored, favored when you receive a little something extra from the Lord, a bonus, not because you did anything to deserve it, but because God out of His agape love just wanted to give it to you.

Our love for each other was so obvious that even as Ernest referred to them, our "naysayers" saw it. At work, my co-worker Debbie told me, "Girl you're dancing around here like you're 16 years old." She was tickled to see me so happy.

At Voorhees Dialysis Center, they said, "Man you're just grinning and not fussing like you used to when things go wrong."

Of course, everybody wasn't happy with us or for us. Many snickered, criticized, questioned and talked negatively about our relationship. Ernest said at the onset, "Let me be the one to tell people at C.C.U about us," and I did. Thank God we listened to His voice and our hearts and didn't allow the naysayers to steal our joy.

When we shared our love with our children, they gave us their full support and blessings. They only wanted us to be happy. Ernest told me when his youngest son, Ernie, came to visit (even before our relationship) when he introduced me to him he asked him, "Son what about her?"

His son responded, "She's OK dad. Stay away from those young girls. They might kill you."

I had to tell my nurse manager in case I ever had to work at Voorhees. I could not care for Ernest or even work on the same side of the room where he was getting his treatment. There had been previous relationships with staff and patients of this manner. While not encouraged, it did happen, and this was the policy.

Ernest was so excited! He couldn't keep it to himself. He told staff and patients alike who his "baby" was and who he was going to marry.

Soon the word got to my unit at Washington Township Dialysis, Every unkind word and negative attitude just drew us closer to each other and God. We either prayed about it or laughed about it.

One of the things we really got a running joke about was when I called my childhood friend, who was like a sister to me. She promoted herself to sister when my one and only sister, Dorothy, passed away suddenly on October 6,1999. During our telephone visit, I shared with her my love for Ernest and our plans to marry.

Naturally she wanted to know **all** about him. I casually informed her that he was a bilateral amputee, wheelchair dependent, had peripheral vascular disease, he'd had 8 heart attacks, and had been married 4 times.

She exclaimed, "Oh, my God, my sister is on crack!"

So, when I mentioned to Ernest that I had told my close friend about his medical condition and what her response was, we both had a good laugh. But, we knew others, whether they said it out loud, whispered it among themselves, had pillow talks about it or just reflected in their own minds, thought the same thing.

When I wrote to my cousin Roger, who was incarcerated at the time, he was happy for me. So much so that from the New York State Penitentiary he ordered stuffed puppy dogs, a boy and girl kissing on a red heart-shaped pillow, to be delivered to my house. When I received it, I took it over to Ernest's room when he was in Manor Care. It followed him to the Kennedy Health Care Center until his death.

It is now on my dresser, right next to the lovely keepsake box Klisa made for me after Ernest's death. Ernest loved and appreciated it the kissing puppy dogs and so did I. We kept it placed in an area where we could glance up at it daily. Thank you again Roger X Powell from the bottom of my heart.

"Come Clean'

Ernest asked me about a month into our relationship, "Tell me what attracted you to me? I'm not that handsome. I have no money; my sole income is a social security disability check for $970.00 a month. I live in a low income, one-bed room senior citizen apartment. I'm in a wheelchair with no legs. The sex may never happen because my wee-wee is out of whack because of the diabetes and history of high blood pressure and will probably never work again."

My answer, "I watched you all those years and saw you as a Man of God, not so much as a preacher. You could have been a janitor, but I saw a Man of God. *1 Timothy 6:11-12"* says it so beautifully. In my own words 'a Man of God is not perfect, he is not God, but he loves God, he has faith in God, he is humble, he loves the word of God, he is a man of prayer, he is not ashamed to share the word of God and purposes to live by it.' Even you, Ernest W. Lewis, when you're tired, in pain, feeling totally wiped out from chronic diarrhea, you Ernest pressed your way to lift up the name of Jesus. You are THAT handsome.

"I don't care about your money. I have no problem coming here to live. This is so convenient and comfortable for you. I'll just have to rent a storage space nearby for my personal belongings. I don't see you as a man in a wheelchair. I see you as a Man of God. I just dream of snuggling up close to you in bed during the day and all night long." That's where his nickname, "snuggles," came from.

We shared our nicknames with Minister Ian and Debbie Simmons at Mom Hamilton's 90th birthday party. It was held at the VFW in Williamstown on July 10, 2010. We sat at the same table. Ernest was "snuggles" to me, and I remember the love letter he wrote, I was "precious to him." That's when we went more public with our relationship for those at C.C.U. who didn't know we were a couple.

We sat close to each other. I made his plate when the food was served, and we left together. He told me later that night that one of the male church members whispered in his ear, "You know Sis. Howard lives right across the street."

He said he told him, "I know!"

We did find out that New Jersey transit did stop just a block away from where I lived. Indeed, he could come whenever he pleased. He was using his prosthesis then and could walk up the 5 steps to my front door.

Our Weekend

The McMillan family reunion, on my father's side, takes place the last weekend of July. We rotate sites. This year it was in North Carolina. I had made plans to go. Ernest's niece was getting married in Michigan and Lucy, his sister, had made arrangements to drive.

She invited Ernest to join her and her son Josh. He accepted. When he told me what weekend it was, I realized that it was the same weekend as my family reunion. I laughed and told him. "You know those busy bodies at C.C.U. When they don't see us in church, they are going to think we went away together."

He laughed and said, "You know, you're right."

I had already mentioned to a few people that I would be away that weekend. Ernest asked me to drive him to his sister's house in Philadelphia. That would make it a little easier for them to hit the highway. I was a little nervous about driving, but more excited about the prospect of us being together on a drive and having a chance to meet his sister and nephews. This would be our first, and not knowing then, our last drive together.

I arrived at Ernest's apartment as scheduled. I learned quickly that he had a very low tolerance for tardiness. I grabbed his suitcase and he rode in his manual chair. The motorized chair, which of course he preferred, was too heavy to take. As we were leaving, lo and behold, we ran into the C.C.U. senior housing gang hanging out in the lobby.

One of the residents greeted me with a smile and said, "Oh, that's right. You did say you were going away for the weekend."

Thank God for the Holy Spirit that constrains us. I simply responded, "Yes, I did." *Luke 12:11, 12.*

When we got to the car Ernest said, "Let them think what they want. We know and God knows we're not going away together." Ernest then proceeded to use his GPS on his cell phone to get us to Lucy's house. Thank God! I was born and raised in Philadelphia, but where Lucy lived seemed like it was out of the city limits.

When we got there, they were just about ready to pull out. We chatted a little and loaded up the van with Ernest's stuff then Lucy gave me excellent directions to get back to Jersey. Before they pulled off, Ernest gave me a CD.

As soon as I got back home, I was missing him already. I pulled out the CD and saw it was titled "Love Songs Just 4 U" from "Snuggles to Precious." Of course, I immediately played it. It started off with a sermon then the song "I Won't Complain." Oh how beautiful! Then love songs for the "baby boomers." I called him and said, "You would have me here listening to these love songs when you are so far away. You are cruel!"

He responded, "I was hoping you would like them."

That night, Dr. Millicent Thompson Hunter, the author of *Don't Die In The winter, Pot Liquor,* and *Crashing Satan's Party*, was coming to our church. I thanked God that my flight was not until the next morning. She and Rev. Goldstein were prayer partners. I had once sent a love and thank you note by Rev. Goldstein to her for how blessed and inspired I was by her books. She was gracious enough to respond back with a note. Dr. Thompson-Hunter was gracious enough to autograph my books that I had brought with me to service.

I made a point of arriving early anticipating a big crowd. Who did I run into but the resident from C.C.U. senior housing.

The resident was shocked to see me, and said, "I thought you were going away?"

I responded, "Yes, my flight leaves in the morning."

Ain't God good? He will fight your battles if you just keep still. When I got home after the service, I called Ernest and told him what happened. We both had a good laugh!

Trouble in Paradise

When I reflect on this episode, I still feel badly. When I arrived in North Carolina, my cell phone battery was low. I did manage to call Ernest and let him know I had arrived safely.

When I arrived to the hotel, my room wasn't ready. In the meantime, my cell phone went dead. When I got to my room, it was more like a suite. It was beautiful! I immediately plugged in my phone to recharge it and went out to join in with all the activities.

When I returned to my room, it was late and I was tired. I fell asleep without calling Ernest. When I awoke the next morning, I was in a panic because I realized I never called him that evening. When I checked my phone, I had about 10 messages from him. Boy was he mad. I found out later he had even called my children because he was so worried about me.

I took a deep breath and nervously called him. Like I said, boy was he mad. I apologized.

He kept saying, "We always call each other and say good night." I just wanted to dig a hole and bury myself in it. I was so upset and I just burst out into tears. He then realized how sincere I was and calmed down. He said, "You owe me. You owe me big time."

I timidly responded, "When we get back to Jersey, can I pay you in installments?"

I was learning that because of his physical limitations and experiencing unfaithful relationships in the past, he needed to feel he had full control. He said on more than one occasion, "I need you to respect me as the authority." My love for him made it easy for me to give him that position and support his decisions with prayer.

Take a Chance

Ernest, at this time had been on dialysis about 10 years. He had come to a point that every dialysis patient fears, he had run out of accesses. He wasn't a candidate for peritoneal dialysis, his chronic diarrhea made the risk of infection too great. He wasn't a candidate for a kidney transplant because of his overall medical history, including several heart attacks, diabetes, peripheral vascular disease, and other health issues.

He had failed vascular accesses in his arm and chest perm caths and had been advised not to have one placed in his thigh. He had a left groin perm cath , the only option left. This limited him. At times, it was uncomfortable because of its position. He couldn't take a tub bath or shower. If the dressing got wet, he could become infected, which would necessitate changing the catheter or replacing it.

He wanted so badly to have another "shot" at getting a vascular access. He sought another surgeon who assured him that he could place a vascular access, namely a graft in his right thigh. These accesses were quite common, so he wanted to go for it.

When he discussed it with me, he had already made up his mind. I reminded him from my experience that I had seen perm caths in patients last for years and that he was getting good flows and clearances from the one he had. But as he reminded me, the decision ultimately was his.

We prayed that God would guide the surgeon's hand and that this access would be successful. The Sunday before his surgery, Rev. Poulson preached a sermon that truly blessed him and he was encouraged to forge ahead. On August 19, 2010, he went to another hospital outside of the Kennedy System where he dialyzed and had a right thigh graft placed in same-day surgery.

I had to work that day, but when I got off, I called to see if he was still there at the hospital. I was told he was. I hurriedly went home, showered, dressed in his favorite color and went to be there when he was discharged.

When I arrived, he was still in the operating room because he was a later case. So, I waited. He had no idea I was there, so I asked the receptionist to let me know when he reached the recovery room, and she did.

When I had been there for several hours, I guess she felt sorry for me and asked if he knew I was coming, I told her, "No. I wanted to surprise him." She called and got permission for me to go up and see him in recovery.

I thanked her, she said, "I didn't want him to be discharged and leave, since he didn't know you were coming." I thanked her again.

After gowning up when I entered the recovery room his face lit up like a Christmas tree. Boy was he surprised. The staff started greeting me, "You must be Precious. How in the world did he get a name like Snuggles?" He had told them all about us. This is something that he continued to do whenever he got a chance to share our love story.

Ernest went home by ambulance because of his motorized wheelchair; I would pick up dinner and meet him at his apartment. I was so happy. My baby was a little sore, but everything went well with the surgery and he was coming home.

I stopped by one of our soon-to-be regulars; Subway, and got him his usual meatball marinara with extra sauce on flat bread. I got a veggie patty on flat bread. It had been a long day for both of us and we just ate half of our sandwiches and he said he needed to lie down.

I helped him get settled, gave him a couple of pain pills and he dozed off. I stretched out on his sofa in the living room. I decided to spend the night; I was off the next day, to be there just in case he needed anything.

He awoke a few hours later and when I heard him moaning, I went in to check on him. Again, he was surprised. "You're still here? What time is it?" I then told him I decided to stick around just in case he needed something.

He said, "Well, since you're still here, you might as well jump in the bed with me."

I hesitated, and he said, "I'm in too much pain to even think about it, you're safe."

I got him a couple of more pain pills and eased into bed with him so as not to disturb his new incision. I was so happy just to be lying in the bed with him. About 4 a.m., he awoke in a panic. It was his dialysis day and his ambulance came between 4:30 and 4:45. He rushed and got in his motorized wheelchair, went into the bathroom, got washed up and dressed. He instructed me to "stay put" until he left with the ambulance drivers and to lock up when I left, which I did.

Since our relationship started in June, I often frequented his apartment. It was easier because it was so handicapped prepared. We would order out, watch TV, and he showed me his photo albums. We also watched videos, and did eventually watch "The Book of Eli," but it really didn't hold his interest so we just talked. He had so many stories about his very colorful past. My life was so boring compared to his.

His neighbors were very much in tune with my comings and goings. One approached me and told me how "nice" it was that I was seeing Rev. Lewis and spending so much time with him. When I told Ernest, he told me her apartment was on the first floor facing the parking lot.

I began becoming increasingly concerned about his new access. He still was having a lot of pain. While he had a strong bruit, a sign that he had good blood flow, he had a disposable stethoscope and we checked it daily. It was warm and red, and I suggested he call the surgeon. He said he would wait a while.

After another day or two, I offered to call the surgeon for him. He firmly told me he would take care of it. Six days after his access was placed, he called me at work and told me to come right over when I got off. He was going to the hospital.

I arrived and he told me what to pack for him to take. It was something I would become accustomed to doing on his frequent trips to the ER. He pulled the emergency cord in his apartment and called 911 and said, "Don't you say anything. Let me do the talking."

When they arrived, he told them he had chest pain. He wanted them to transport him to the hospital that placed the thigh graft. They informed him that with his complaint of chest pain, he had to go to the nearest hospital. He was able to persuade them to take him to Kennedy Stratford Division.

He told me to go to Monday night prayer and then meet him at the hospital. I begged him to let me follow him to Stratford, insisting, "They don't need me at prayer; I want to be with you." He said OK.

Stratford was very familiar to him. He had been there many times as an outpatient and inpatient because of its close proximity to his dialysis unit. He was all too familiar with the staff.

One person in particular, he always looked forward to seeing was Joe Gatero, who started out as a volunteer that checked in on patients when they came in through the ER and in-patients to see if they had any concerns or needs during their stay. He became such a valuable asset to Kennedy that they created a paying position for him.

Ernest met Joe several years ago. I believe it was the time he had a severe reaction to Cipro. This was an antibiotic that literally made him lose his mind. His confusion was so great that he required hospitalization and was never able to remember what transpired during that stay. He told me he was dating a lady at that time and he said some things to her that made her break off their relationship, none of which he could remember.

Joe came to check on him daily and remembered from previous hospitalizations that he enjoyed reading the newspaper. Joe brought him the paper every day until he was back to normal. He said when he finally became more lucid; he had a whole stack of papers in his room and he knew his friend Joe had been there.

Ernest was admitted and treated with antibiotics, and once he was stabilized about a week to 10 days later he was then transferred to the hospital that placed the right thigh graft. They took him to the OR and removed the infected graft. In the recovery room he saw the same nurses who were there when the access was placed. They remembered my nickname and struggled with his until they finally got it.

This hospital had its perks, I was not an employee so I couldn't come and go as I pleased, but their visiting hours lasted until 11 pm and their private rooms were so big and beautiful. He usually had a private room because of the diarrhea, so we still had plenty of time to spend together. Once stable after the graft was removed he was ready for Rehab. Yippee!

On September 28, 2010, he called me at work and said he was being transferred to Meadowview that evening. I didn't go to Bible study that night. I wanted to be there to help him get settled. Meadowview was so close to where I lived; not even a 10-minute drive. I was so grateful.

He kept calling with updates. Ambulance transportation, we both knew, could be so frustrating. As it started getting late, I decided I'd better just go and wait because I wasn't sure what the visiting hours were.

As soon as the ambulance arrived he called me. I told him, "I'm right here." I just followed them in when they took Ernest. I went with them to his room and started putting away his belongings. When the nurse and nursing assistant came to help get him in bed, the nurse was quite annoyed, informing me that visiting hours were over.

Ernest quickly spoke up and said, "She's my fiancé and she's only trying to help me get situated."

We had established early in our relationship always to have each other's back in public. If we disagreed, we would do that privately. If he wanted me to be quiet, he would squeeze my hand. If I wanted him to calm down, I would stroke his hand.

As they were transferring him into the bed, we noticed some bloody drainage on his right thigh where he had the surgery. The nurse did not like the look of it and wanted to send him back to the hospital. Ernest insisted his dressing was dry when he left and felt maybe with the move and ambulance ride the wound leaked a little. She reinforced it and said she would return later and check on it. I left soon afterwards.

We were so happy. Again he was in a private room, and still close by for our daily visits.

Movie Scene

The next morning about 7a.m., I received a phone call at work. It was Meadowview. The nurse had found Ernest in a pool of blood and he was being rushed to the hospital. She said he was alert and being taken to Kennedy.

I asked which Division. She said, "Washington Township."

I said, "Thank God." It was right across the street. I had just a few more meds to pass out and informed one of the nurses that I was taking my break, and that I was leaving the building.

As I was running across the street, I was still thanking God that he was so close. I stopped at the ER reception desk to find out what room he was in. Being in uniform with my Kennedy name badge, I was able to easily go to his room without question.

As Ernest so often relived that day, it was like something from a movie scene. His room was so crowded I couldn't even get in to let him know I was there. I just stood outside the door and listened as intently as I could to find out what was going on.

He was bleeding from his femoral artery. There was a young doctor on his right holding pressure, and the others were barking orders for labs, IV fluids, trying to get a central line placed, watching his vital signs and level of consciousness. They were giving orders for stat type and cross, and a need for the OR.

Like Ernest so often said, "It was WILD!"

After a few minutes, the drama calmed down. They got a central line in for IV fluids, the young doctor was still applying pressure, and labs had been drawn and sent stat so everybody was able to take a deep breath. The room started to clear out and that's when I made my way up to the head of the stretcher and he knew I was there.

Now those remaining were staring at me and Ernest said, "You see this beautiful black woman, this is my fiancé." He knew it embarrassed me every time he said it, but he said it anyway.

I told him how much I loved him, and prayed for him, then I told him, "I have to go back to work, but that I would return as soon as possible."

I went straight to my nurse manager's office and told her what was going on. She said, "Lydia go! Get your things and go. I'll get someone to come in and take your assignment." I ran and got my things and left not saying a word to anyone.

When I returned, I learned the plan was emergency surgery to patch up the artery. Blood had been ordered and they were only waiting for an available operating room.

I asked Ernest who he wanted me to call and he told me, "As long as I am alert, I'll tell you who to call and what information I want them to have. If I ever get to the point I can't tell you, I'm sure by then you'll know who to call and what to say. Call Rev. Hargrove, my sisters and my sons. That's all for now." He then asked the nurse to give me his personal belongings and told me all his numbers were in his cell phone.

I called Rev. Hargrove first and he said he would be right over. Ernest then told me I could call the others later. He just wanted to talk. I pulled up a stool and we did just that. We talked of the love that God had given us for the past 3 months. We talked about how happy we had made each other.

The young doctor was still there holding pressure to his right artery, but we didn't care. We were professing our love like we were alone. I told him, "When God brings you through this, I'm going to move in with you. I don't care how much people talk."

He said, "You'd do that for me?"

I answered, "Yes, that and even more." He told me I had been better to him than all his other wives put together.

Rev. and Sister Hargrove arrived and had prayer. They instructed me to call if I needed anything. Rev. Hargrove told me to call when the surgery was done no matter how late it was.

When we relived that day, which we did several times, Ernest said, "Pastor and Sister Hargrove really thought I was checking out that time, didn't they?"

I said, "I think they did, too."

The surgeon was getting angry and frustrated. The OR had not called back about a room. She said, "Let's go. Tell them I'm on my way and they better have a room ready or I'm going to lose him."

With the young doctor still holding on, the surgeon pulling the stretcher and another doctor pushing, away they went with me walking quickly on the side. The ER nurse, seeing me, said, "You can't go."

The surgeon said, "Leave her alone, let's go."

Then the ER nurse screamed out, "What about your purse?"

I screamed back, "I don't care about my pocketbook."

As we were rolling down the hall, Ernest was telling me to tell his sisters and sons how much he loved them. Ernest said, *"You have to tell the story."*

I replied, "I can't tell it as well as you."

Then he repeated, *"You have to tell the story."*

I, holding on to hope, asked him what paper he wanted, I brought him the newspaper every day, rotating between the *Philadelphia Inquirer* and the *Courier Post*. He said, "Both."

By that time we were outside the OR and I said, "You got it. I love you so much!" Then they rolled him through the door.

The Wait

I was now at my wit's end, not knowing where to go next. I decided to go to the acute dialysis unit hoping and praying that Jasmine was working. Thank God she was. Of course she was aware of what was going on because he was a dialysis patient.

I was trying desperately to hold it together, she was trying to take me to their break room when we heard an overhead page, "Mrs. Lewis, please call —, Mrs. Lewis please call —,"

Jaz, as we call her at work, said, "That call is for you, They think you are his wife." Of course, I wasn't paying any attention to the page. She helped me with the number. She said, "It's probably the Operating Room."

It was them, wanting to know the number on his pacemaker/defibrillator. I told them to call his dialysis unit at Voorhees and that I didn't have that information on me.

They challenged me, "Well, you have his wallet don't you?"

I repeated, "Please call the Voorhees unit." Jaz agreed to let them call Voorhees.

Jaz insisted I go to the break room and stay as long as I needed and she would come back and check on me .She still had patients in the unit. I used that time to first call his sisters Brenda and Lucy, ex-wife Sherrill and then his sons, Marcus and Ernie. We cried and prayed together.

I then started calling the prayer warriors. Bonnie, the secretary from church, called me and offered to come over and she gave me her cell phone number. I reassured her I was OK right now. *Liar, Liar, pants on fire.*

I paced the floor. I asked Jaz for Sylvia's phone number because I couldn't even remember Leona, my daughter, or my son Leon's cell phone numbers. Jaz kept running back and forth checking on me. I thank God so much even as I write this for that.

She kept trying to get me to eat. She forced me to take her orange and she said I could always eat it later. I confided in her later that I did eat it about 10 days later and it was as sweet and juicy as could be. Now I have a new appreciation for oranges.

After about two hours, I decided to go to the surgical waiting room. This time I had more clout. The surgeons knew I would be waiting to hear some news. I checked in and gave them my cell phone number.

In the meantime, I was receiving calls on my phone and Ernest's cell from his family because they didn't have my number. Then I drifted down to the chapel and fell before the altar and confessed I was being selfish, but I just wanted him to stay here a little while longer. I paced the tiny chapel floor and was up and down on my knees. In exasperation I would leave, walk around the hospital, cell phones in hand not wanting to miss any calls, and return to the surgical waiting room to check for updates.

When I returned to the chapel that afternoon, I found an elderly lady there praying. We acknowledged each other and continued to pray silently to ourselves. We both were there for hours. When my cell phone rang, I respectfully left and took the call, and then returned to pray or just meditate. Then a younger lady came in and approached the elderly lady and said "he's OK, we can go up and see him now."

The older lady as she left smiled and said, "God bless you."

That's when I had my meltdown. I screamed softly to myself, "God, I have been here much longer than she. I've been on my knees. She's so old, she probably can't even get down on her knees and she's gotten the answer that her loved one is OK and she can go up to see him." I boo-hooed and cried, "I can't take this. You think I'm strong but I'm not."

Pacing the floor even more frantically, I said, "I have to talk to somebody!" I started to call Bonnie, but then I thought she's still finishing up at work, so I called Debbie, my sister, my friend, my co-worker at the dialysis unit.

Debbie knows the Lord. She loves the Lord. What I felt I needed was just a hug, not a whole lot of church jargon; not a scripture quoting, Bible toting sistah. Just an old-fashioned hug that said "I'm here for you, sistah." Not a "let me preach to you sistah." Not a "let me sing you a gospel hymn, sistah." Just, "if you want to cry your eyes out go right ahead I'm here for you, sistah." I pulled out my staff phone number list; we all have it in case we want to switch days, and called.

When she heard my weeping voice, she said, "What's wrong?" I was crying so hard I could hardly tell her. She then said, "Where are you?"

I answered, "In the chapel at Kennedy."

She said, "I'll be right over." She came, wearing a baseball cap, sweats and sneakers and I flooded the chapel with my tears. I thank God for Debbie because she allowed me to be myself. She sat there and let me get it all out. We even laughed when I told her about the old lady's prayer being answered before mine.

Thank you Debbie from the bottom of my heart. A friend is always loyal, and "a brother is born to help in time of need" (*Proverbs 17:17*). She later told me that she and her son were outside raking leaves. When I called, her husband answered the phone and said, "It's Miss Lydia, something's wrong."

Back to the surgical waiting room, still no word. So I just decided to wait. The receptionist as she was leaving for the day assured me it would be OK for me to stay. I was the only one there. She knew I had been there all day and so graciously gave me a meal ticket for the hospital cafeteria. I tried to decline, but she insisted I take it, "You need to go and get something to eat. It's been a long day."

I thanked her, and after the elevator door closed I waited a few minutes and tore up the meal ticket. How could anyone think I would want anything to eat at a time like this, when my Ernest had been in the OR all day long?

Yes, I was angry and I recognized how ungrateful I was but I didn't care. I was angry and scared. I found myself pacing the floor again, back and forth, going around chairs in a circle until I was exhausted.

I could feel myself getting dehydrated and sat down and drank the bottle of water I had brought with me. Then I started the pacing again. I noticed the Keurig machine and after messing up a few cups, I finally got the hang of it. I made myself a cup of lemon zinger tea. It was quite delicious and calming.

I started repenting for my poor attitude over the past few hours and I felt God was telling me, "OK, missy, for that little temper tantrum you threw about me answering the old lady's prayer before yours, you just made your wait longer."

It was late when the surgeons came to the waiting room, maybe 8 or 9 p.m. The two came in looking somber and exhausted. The chief surgeon applauded the resident for the fine job she did, stating she tried everything. That's why the surgery was so long. She tried to patch up the artery with one of his natural vessels, but he had none. They repaired it with a synthetic material and were hoping his body would not reject it and that it would hold up.

The chief surgeon was amazed that Ernest, with all of his health problems, was not only still here, but had an independent and social lifestyle. He warned me that he was not out of the woods yet and as I very well knew, the first 48 hours were crucial.

Even with his reservations, I thanked God for the both of them. I told the attending surgeon I was trusting God to bring him through. He just nodded and walked away. I called Rev. Hargrove and gave him the good news. "He made it!"

The Awakening

Like I said earlier, Ernest shared with me so many stories, and so much of his life before we met. I felt honored and privileged when he told me many of them he had never told anyone else, not even his other wives or girlfriends.

We just felt so comfortable with each other that we talked about everything together. That's what I really miss our talks. Often he would say, "Can we mute the TV and just talk?" He would tell me about his day when I would go over right after work and I would share mine.

I would call him on my breaks and before I pulled out of the parking lot, he would call me at work and sing "I love you for sentimental reasons" and I would respond, "I love you for all kinds of reasons."

When he called me at work no matter how busy it was I was revitalized when he so often would say, "Who loves you baby?"

I would respond, "Jesus and you."

Or when he would just call and sing, "I just called to say I love you."

I would call him sometimes and say, "Hey, handsome, what are you wearing?"

He would answer, "A T-shirt and diaper, come on down!" Then we both would laugh.

Yes we had romance in "spite of" the kind most dream of and so many have never had. WE WERE BLESSED AND HIGHLY FAVORED!

He shared his previous marriages. His first to Sherrill, his high school sweetheart, December 25, 1968, then Peggy, December 11, 1975, then Deborah, November 29,1987, and his present to Brenda, June 29, 1990.

He talked often of his children, Marcus Wayne, his oldest from his marriage with Sherrill, Ruby that he was told he fathered while stationed in Germany, Vanessa and Erick from his relationship with Cherry Ann, and Ernest, 11, his son from his marriage with Brenda.

He loved his children and his wives' children from previous marriages and relationships. He made every attempt to be a father as long as his wives or girlfriends allowed it. Whenever he talked of Brenda, he always differentiated Brenda the sister or Brenda the wife. I never met any of them until that night.

As I waited for Ernest to be transferred from recovery to the ICU unit Sherrill, Ernest's first wife arrived. I had called her and with one of the conversations I had with

Marcus their son, he asked if his mom had come. I told him I didn't know and that I really didn't know what she looked like. She came into the waiting room and introduced herself. I updated her on Ernest's status and we waited together.

When he arrived and had gotten settled, the nurse came and escorted us to the room. The nurse glanced at us both, trying to decide to whom she should be giving the update. I sensed her hesitation and explained, "She is the ex-wife and I am the fiancé."

Ernest had various IV pumps all around him and was intubated. He opened his eyes, looked and saw Sherril and me at the foot of the bed and then closed his eyes.

Days later, he shared, "When I woke up and saw the two of you together, I thought, 'Oh Crap!' and I just closed my eyes." We all had a good laugh.

Ernest bounced back rather quickly, he extubated himself the next day even with mitts in place. He told me then "don't let them put that thing down my throat again" and made that part of his living will/advanced directive. The diarrhea persisted with 10 to 20 stools a day and that really drained him.

Wedding Plans

On ctober 4, 2010, feeling that he had turned the corner, we started making wedding plans. We thought about returning to Winslow Diner for our reception. They did have a small area that we could use. We started our guest list that consisted of relatives, Prayer Warriors and a few others from the church, and a few from dialysis.

We also discussed songs. I chose "At Last" by Etta James. He liked that choice too, and said, "Maybe we can get her to come out of retirement and sing at our wedding."

I said that would be nice. I also favored "When I Found You" by BeBe Winans that Herb sang to Tonya at their wedding, a young couple from our church. Ernest was interested.

He said, "Maybe I can get the words and learn the melody and sing it to you."

We talked about going away for a short honeymoon. Somewhere he could get dialysis. I told him I would love to go to New York to see the places he lived, the schools he attended, the corners "he hung out on" and the churches he attended and preached at.

We were excited and happy and moving ahead with his divorce and getting married. During that time he gave me all his banking information, including his pin # to his debit card. I wrote out his checks for his apartment and all his bills.

Of course I had the keys to his apartment and to his mailbox. He shared this with a close friend, who questioned his trust. He told me his response to the friend was "If she runs off with that little bit I have, it will never come close to all that she has given to me."

I loved Ernest and my goal in life with him after seeing and hearing about all the pain and suffering he endured was to make him happy and comfortable. That's something I told him more times than I can remember, "I just want you to be happy and comfortable."

I had no intention of taking anything from him. Not even his role of leadership. Thank God he saw that early in our relationship and defended me when anyone else insinuated otherwise!

The Operating Room Again

The synthetic graft did not hold up. Ernest started to get decreased blood flow to his right leg, so back to the OR he went on October 10, 2010 for a revision. Brenda his sister had driven up from Michigan. She and her son, Jason, and grandson, Joshua, accompanied her. Yes, they do surgery on Sunday.

We met at the hospital, Brenda, Sherrill and I, that morning, spent time with Ernest and had prayer. After he left for the OR, we decided to go to C.C.U. and have dinner. The church was serving dinner that day. Afterwards we returned to the hospital. Don't judge me, God knows his children. When I couldn't sit one minute longer listening or joining in with small talk, I would excuse myself and pace outside the elevator or run up and down the three flights of steps to the ground floor.

It was during this time that I started to let my guard down with Sherrill. Sherril told Brenda and me how Ernest had prayed for someone to come into his life. Someone who understood him and could handle his illness and be there for him and with him. She said he had found that person in me. Sherrill also said how happy she was for him that I, a dialysis nurse, was perfect for him.

That marked the beginning of our sister friendship that is still intact today. Ernest had told me so much about her. I knew her as his high school sweetheart, mother of his first born and best friend for over 40 years.

When Sherrill came to visit, they had so much in common, they shared so much history that I felt like an outsider looking in. They talked and laughed about old friends, old times, old places that I knew nothing of. I felt left out.

He once said to me after one of Sherrill's visits, "You were just sitting there smiling. Why didn't you just jump in and join us in the conversation?"

I told him, "You were talking about things I didn't have any idea about."

Then he assured me that Sherrill had all the respect in the world for me, that I had nothing to fear from her and that she would always be his son's mother and his friend. "We've been through a lot together, but we both know we will never get back together."

When Sherrill and I were together to visit Ernest, he made a point of introducing us as, "This is Sherrill, my first wife, and this is Lydia, my fiancé and my last wife." People would marvel and say this is the way it should be with past and present relationships.

Rehab Again

After multiple trips back to the OR for incision and drainage and revisions, which totaled about 23, he was deemed ready for rehab. By this time, he was really beat up. That last surgery really took a toll; so much scar tissue, lumps and bumps on his right abdomen. He was sent to Manor Care Fries Mills on November 9, 2011 with a wound vac in place for the last area to heal.

Thank God for working in the nursing profession. One of my patient's husband told us of a brand new Rehab that was opened on Fries Mills Road, not far from the hospital. So I requested he be sent there. The facility was beautiful. It was a nicely decorated, state of the art building. The rooms were so big and nicely furnished.

When he first arrived, Ernest quite frankly was intimidated by the size. It was so big and the beds had no side rails, which would be a challenge for a weak bilateral amputee. He had no roommate, of course, because of the chronic diarrhea. The Clostridium Difficile would clear up and then resume and he would again have 10 to 20 stools a day.

But I was there. There was no restriction with visitation. If you came at a time the facility was locked, you rang a bell, identified yourself and were granted a visit. With Ernest being in the room alone, our visits would not infringe or disturb the privacy of a roommate.

One of the staff told me, "Girl we need to get you a swipe card or a key so you can come and go as you please without bothering us with ringing that bell."

I thank God that through the two years and 2 months of being in one facility or another, that I was there every day except when he made me go to Israel, when I had and evening CPR class that I didn't get out until very late, when I had a routine colonoscopy and was not allowed to drive for 24 hours, and Hurricane Sandy.

He insisted I not change my church activities. One Sunday when I came to visit after going to an afternoon service, he told me this one Sunday, "I wished you disobeyed me, skipped that service and came straight here. I really needed you to just hold my hand." My heart ached .

After that, I stopped attending the afternoon services and just went to the morning ones. Oh how I was criticized for being with him so much. But thank God, I listened to GOD and my heart. We both knew with all that lovey-dovey stuff that we shared, that our days together were numbered and we were determined to be with each other as long as God allowed!

My mother often sang a song, "Nobody knows the trouble I see, nobody knows but Jesus." Nobody knew how often he had to be changed, nobody knew how long he was left in dirty diapers and a soiled bed, and nobody knew the nasty attitudes and unkind remarks of staff that cared for him. ONLY God, Ernest and me.

What they didn't know was quite often because of the pain medication and fevers, he became confused and often hallucinated. Ernest appreciated the fact that I was there to fill in the blanks for him and the nursing staff did, too. He told me so often how grateful he was when he would doze off and awake and see me by his side reading, watching TV, taking a snooze with him or just holding his hand.

Deacon Carter encouraged me by saying, "Sis don't pay any attention to what others think or say, you know what you have to do."

Like I said, I wanted Ernest to be happy and comfortable. So I made myself available. The staff quickly learned that and when I came they knew he would be well taken care of. I knew it was frustrating for the staff as well as for him. As soon as he would eat, it would come out of him in large amounts so quickly that you couldn't even place a bedpan under him even if you had one, you definitely did not have time to get him on a commode. So to ease their burden when I was there I would clean and change him.

You know that saying, "He's not heavy, he's my brother." They knew when I came I didn't mind taking care of him.

One CNA told Ernest, "She does it out of love." Yes it was not even a labor of love, just love.

Staff in the nursing home would often say, "He's so lucky to have someone like you in his life."

I would respond, "We are both blessed, this is not a one sided relationship."

They could see our love and commitment to each other was just as strong if not stronger than those who are married. We were both blessed. Often when I would come over after work, he would tell me, "Sit down, take off your shoes and socks," Then he would proceed to massage my feet or tell me to sit on the side of the bed so he could massage my neck and shoulders.

We endeavored to make one another feel loved and special. With all those diaper and bed changes, I made every effort to maintain his dignity and we even made light of it. We joked and laughed as I cleaned him.

Early on, we even nicknamed his private parts. It was nothing dirty, vulgar, or obscene. It was words that an **innocent** five year old would say. Some of you may be thinking, "come on Lydia, that's just too much information."

Allow me to share with you how our intimate relationship blessed so many others. In this world there are literally millions of couples because of illness, medication, or just age can no longer perform sexually.

We've learned, as hopefully others have or will, that couples can still maintain a sense of intimacy with the way they interact with one another. It can be a glance, a touch, or a word. You have noticed I have referred to Rev. Lewis throughout this book as Ernest. At the onset of our relationship, he told me that I was his woman, not his nurse, not his missionary, not his evangelist, but his woman.

When he was in the hospital, rehab, or nursing home he insisted when referring to him that I call him Ernest, not Rev. Lewis. He said they knew he was a Reverend; he had a number of his certificates, licenses and ordination papers on the wall, so referring to him as Rev. was not necessary.

When a man and woman are in love and have made a lifetime commitment to one another there is still a need to satisfy one another sexually. That's the way God made us. When men still desire to make their woman "feel like a natural woman," "girl you're one hot mama" and a woman still desires to make her man feel like a macho man, you make my toes curl man," we substitute the act of sex with words. That ladies and gentleman is how you maintain that intimacy. We were blessed when others observed this and it opened up their eyes to another form of lovemaking.

We had so much fun together, more than anyone will ever know, just can't and won't (you may not be able to handle it) tell it all. God blessed us so much, just to enjoy each other to love one another and even make one another feel good about ourselves.

Remember the other part of my January prayer that year, addressed poor self-esteem. When Ernest looked me in the eye, he often scolded me for not always looking him in the eye. One day clear out of the blue he said, "You know what I like about you the most? Your cleft lip. I find it to be beautiful."

Nobody in my entire life had ever said that to me. Most people cringed or looked quickly away. He often, as I said before, introduced me as "his beautiful black woman." Ernest rarely texted but one day he texted me at work, "U R So beautiful to Me." Needless to say, that is one text that I will NEVER delete.

Ain't God good! He answered both of my January prayers in less than a year.

Obama For My Man

Ernest enjoyed reading the paper as I mentioned before. I found a Black newspaper, the Philadelphia Tribune at two convenience stores in Sicklerville. I brought one to Ernest and he liked reading it. It only came out on Tuesday, Friday and Sunday.

One day when I was purchasing the Tuesday paper, I spotted what looked like a President Obama blanket near the t-shirts they had on display. I could hardly contain myself.

When I returned Friday, I saw that the blanket was still there. By then, I had some extra money with me, and even before I picked up the paper I picked up the blanket. It was the only one. It was a black and gray fleece, king-sized blanket with a picture of president Obama with his name across the bottom.

It was beautiful! I bought it before Thanksgiving. I couldn't wait until Christmas. He loved it. He took it everywhere he went; dialysis, doctor visits, ER visits, hospital admissions, everywhere. The only time he left without it was when he came home for Thanksgiving. He knew I would keep him warm that night.

I tried to buy more and I asked the owner to order some for me. I even gave her my phone number, but she said she was no longer able to reach the vendor. Ernest relished the fact that no one else he knew had one.

We were strong Obama supporters and financial contributors. Consequently, we received countless photos of the president his family and even their dog BO. I brought them for Ernest and proudly displayed them in his room, visible for all to see. Those who saw the photo gallery speculated that we had a close connection with the president. They were right. We not only held him and his family up in prayer but supported the Democratic Party to which he belonged financially. You know "put your money where your mouth is."

Visitors From the Big Apple

One cold Saturday winter evening, Ernest called me at work and asked me to pick us up something good for dinner. He was feeling good and looked forward to us just "chilling" out on this Saturday night.

When I arrived he had visitors. Overseer Willie L. Gray and one of her members, Bro. Joshua, had driven from New York on a cold winter's night to visit Ernest. Irene Flores, one of Ernest's friends from New York, had told Overseer Gray about this preacher who had all these surgeries and was now in a rehab facility trying to recover. She came to encourage him.

> *"As we have therefore opportunity,*
> *let us do good unto all men,*
> *especially unto them who are of the household of faith."*
> — Galatians 6:10

Ernest was so elated, I was too that she thought it was not robbery to drive all the way from New York to come, pray and share a word with us. As Ernest, on several occasions said, "We had church." We were so blessed by her presence, prayers, spiritual conversation and personal testimonies. She left her business card and encouraged me to call if we needed anything. Thank You, Overseer Gray. Even preachers need encouragement and they need to know that their co-laborers in the ministry care. We talked of your visit and how you blessed us so many times over and over again.

Overseer Gray's visit was so special not only because she was from his home state, New York where he was born, raised and lived the majority of his life, but she didn't know him. They never met or served together. What a demonstration of love. Rev. Bill Turner also came several times from Delaware to visit and encourage as well as Deacon Rose and an associate minister from his son's church for Bible study and fellowship.

It's been said, "don't stay sick too long" because your support dwindles with each week, month, and in Ernest's case, year that you are away. Just like the marines motto "just a few good men," Ernest was blessed with a handful of men and women who came. called, and visited on a consistent basis — our Pastor and a couple of Ernest's pulpit buddies, you know who you are. He treasured, enjoyed and looked forward to them all.

We knew that there were others, unseen, unsung friends, acquaintances lifting him up in prayer on a regular basis. Those who the Lord led to say a "little prayer" for

Rev. Lewis when he needed it the most. Prayers go where we are unable to go. Ernest was so sweet, so loving even when I wasn't there when he had a visitor he would say, "I love it when they pray for you too, because we're in this together."

Thanksgiving day was quiet, I don't recall any visitors, I went briefly to Leon and Cheryl's where dinner was being served, and I returned to Manor Care with a platter for Ernest and myself and we ate together.

Rehab?

Rehab wasn't easy. Whenever I could, I would meet him when he was doing his exercises and be his cheerleader. "Go Ernest! Go Ernest!" He had so many ER visits and hospital admissions up until December 20th, but he was back at Manor Care for Christmas. My children came over and we celebrated there.

At that visit, my son, Leon, started calling Ernest "Pops" and he was thrilled. He cherished the acceptance, respect and love he felt from my entire family, which included Leon's wife, Cheryl, and their children; Latoya and her husband, Joe; Kenny Wayne; my daughter, Leona, and her husband, Darnell, and son, Lamont. He would often say, "They are so lovable."

He was back in the hospital the 29th of December. New Years Eve, a young doctor came into Ernest's room about 10 p.m. He looked very somber and spoke softly, "Mr. Lewis, I'm sorry to tell you that there is nothing else we can do for you. Your condition has deteriorated and we have run out of treatment options. We have done all we can. I'm sorry, but we have nothing else to offer."

We were speechless. Ernest had been through so much: the surgeries, the chronic diarrhea, bouts of infection, etc. but he was never told that he was at the end of the road. Ernest just said, "Thanks doc," and he left.

We just sat there quietly. It was New Year's Eve. I had bought some plastic flutes, sparkling cider, cheese, veggie cheese and crackers for us to have a little celebration. I had left it in the car and planned to run out and get it when it got closer to midnight.

We just sat there and I could see and feel his pain. I was feeling it, too. He closed his eyes and said, "Excuse me while I take a nap."

I told him, "That's fine." Then, I went to the nurse's station. Ernest had been moved to a room with a patient who also had C. Diff, so I had to respect his roommate's privacy. I couldn't just stay as long as I wanted as I had previously.

I asked the doctor who was at the desk writing if I could stay until after midnight, and he in turn asked one of the nurses. One gave the OK.

Ernest opened his eyes about 11:30 p.m. and I told him I had gotten permission to stay until after midnight. We sat quietly and waited for the "ball" to drop. When midnight came, we started praying. He would pray, then I would pray. Then he would pray and then I would pray.

We continued this until about 12: 45 a.m. and that's when he said, "I will live and not die."

I shall not die, but live and declare the works of the Lord."
— Psalms 118:17

We kissed each other good night said Happy New Year and I left.

I called him the next morning and said, "I'm on my way with breakfast."

He said, "Good, just bring the usual."

When I arrived he said again, "I will live and not die." Then he said, "Didn't that doctor look like he was going to cry last night?"

I said, "He sure did," and we both laughed. I said, "He don't know God the way we do."

"It's not over until God says it's over," Ernest announced. "This year we're going to have Bible study every night, just you and me and I'm going to want you to take the lead sometimes."

I said, "OK, sounds good." And we did. We picked random scriptures and devotionals and prayed and studied God's word together in the evenings after we ate dinner.

I often stayed late with Ernest when I went to visit him to make sure he was comfortable before I left. Even when he was OK, just when I was about to leave he would make some last minute requests, "I'm hungry can you get me a snack?" or "Can you make me a cup of tea?" or "Can you give me a few more minutes? I want to talk." When we finally forced ourselves to separate we would give each other five kisses and then touch our hearts and extend our arms out to each other before I left the room.

On the days that I had to go to work, I would often oversleep. So, he started calling me between 3:30 and 4 a.m. to wake me up. How wonderful it was to hear his voice first thing in the morning.

We would pray together. He would pray for me traveling mercies and a good day at work and I would pray for him less diarrhea, less pain, and on dialysis days a safe and good treatment. When I arrived home after our visit, I would always call to assure him of my safe arrival and sometimes we would talk or pray again.

Oh, how I miss our prayers and talks.

I Messed Up!

On February 9, 2011, Ernest was admitted again, but he was discharged in time for us to celebrate our first Valentine's Day together. Valentine's Day fell on a Monday that year and since Ernest's dialysis treatment was Monday and sometimes he was so drained afterwards, I thought we could celebrate Valentine's Day on Sunday, the day I had off from work and he had off from dialysis.

After church, I called him and said I would treat for dinner. He told me what he wanted and I packed up a basket using the same flutes and sparkling cider from New Year's Eve. Also I brought a CD player, the CD he had given to me in July, two battery operated candles, Valentine's Day paper products and I picked up our dinner from Angelo's.

We watched a little TV and then ate. He was quiet and showed no interest in the music or candles. He said he was tired and wanted to turn in early, so I gave him his card and gifts. I had red t-shirts made with "For God so loved the world" printed on them for both of us.

I also had a sweat shirt, a hoody with the same "For God so loved the world" printed on it for him, and I gave him a red bell with the words ring once for a hug, twice for a kiss. He seemed to like the cards and gifts.

The next day when I got off of work, I went to see him and he told me how so many liked his hoody and all the compliments he had received at dialysis and then he started ringing his "bell." After ringing the bell several times, he told me to go to his closet and get a bag out for him. When I opened the closet door, all these balloons hit me in the face. I said, "Oh, my goodness."

He laughed, and said, "I gotcha!" Yes, he surely did. He stopped me and said, "There's more look in the bottom."

There was more. A beautiful floral arrangement with 12 red roses, one yellow and one white rose, "his signature," a small box of chocolates, and a stuffed animal — a white and pink dog holding a pink heart with the words in red, "Hot 4 U". That is on my dresser today, right beside my keepsake box Klisa made for my "Man of God."

If that wasn't enough he ordered a beautiful heart shaped ruby necklace that you see me wearing today. He ordered dinner, I picked it up and we had a lovely evening.

Two days later, he let me know in no uncertain terms that he was the one to initiate our Valentine's celebration. That I had no right to make the decision to celebrate the day before. That he celebrated holidays on the day, not before and accused me of usurping his authority. I never initiated another holiday or celebration again. I waited for his lead.

Time to Move

Ernest was admitted again on March 14th for a couple of weeks for fluid on the lungs but thanks be to God his wounds were all healed without the need for any more surgery. We were happy and so was his plastic surgeon. He said it was a miracle that those open areas closed up so perfectly without skin grafting. Nothing is too hard for God!

As much as I loved Ernest, his mouth often got him in trouble. He complained so much about the care at Manor Care that when his 100 days were up, they didn't want him to stay. We prayed that he would be placed at Kennedy Health Care Center. It was across the street from where I worked and so close to where I lived.

At the 11th hour, just before I was scheduled to go to Israel, the Lord used a sister in Christ to get him in. They had a long waiting list. We know God can do anything!

I had planned to cancel my trip to the Holy Land but he said no, Sherrill had gone and had come back a different person and I had to go because he would never be able to.

So, I went and he assured me, "I will leave instructions not to do anything until you get back if any thing happens to me while you are gone."

The Holy Land was nothing short of awesome. I am so glad I had that experience. When I returned, I was the one with stories. Oh, so many to tell.

We made plans to go to the Holy Land in Florida the next year. Ernest looked forward to having that experience. I had gone there on our family vacation that Cheryl had arranged in 2009. We as a family planned to return to Florida and we knew that Disney World was handicap accessible and their Holy Land had so much to see and enjoy.

His roommate at Kennedy Health Care Center was Joe and Ernest got a long just fine with him. He was the only one who didn't complain about Joe's almost constant screaming, Joe's wife Jackie appreciated the way Ernest tolerated Joe and that he also looked out for him. They got along well.

We enjoyed a nice vacation from the ER and hospital until 22nd of July where he experienced chest tightness and right shoulder pain. Then, back again 28th of August with fever and chills.

Is This a Problem?

When Ernest was in Manor Care Fries Mills after his wound vac was removed and his wounds were closing up we both felt comfortable with me crawling into bed with him and just snuggling up close together. When one of the CNA's first saw this she jokingly said, "Now, don't you two be making no babies up here."

We would say, "If it's a girl, we'll call her Manorcarette. If it's a boy, Manor Care the 1st."

On the 6 September we found out that the beds in Manor Care were wider or at least they seemed that way. I crawled into bed with Ernest and snuggled up close. We just enjoyed the comfort of being close to one another. When the evening nurse came around with her meds she saw us and just stared. Ernest approached her and asked, "Is this a problem? If so tell me now"

She responded and said, "I'm only concerned about her safety because I don't want her to fall."

Later, the word got back to Ernest that she had informed the nurse manager.

Ernest heard that the nurse manager's response was, "Were they having sex?"

The nurse said, "No. I don't think so."

The nurse manager said, "So what's the problem?"

The nurse manager explained that Ernest was the second youngest resident there. The other being a 50 something male that had been in a motor vehicle accident and was bed bound and had to be fed and didn't talk. Ernest's situation was unique!

Reality Check

Kennedy Health Care Center (KHCC) was asking for all of Ernest's disability check except $35.00 which was for his own personal use. That made it impossible for him to hold on to his apartment. We planned to marry anyway, so the decision was to let the apartment go. We would find handicap accessible housing.

I went over every week and packed up and moved his personal belongings. Some things I stored in my shed. The other things I stored in the house. We decided to sell his furniture and what we did not sell, we would give away. He was so depressed. We decided to put the move to South Carolina on hold and spend another year here after we got married.

Ernest had preached a few times in South Carolina and really liked the country. He was so serious about relocating that he asked me to call Judy and David Shell who lived in Grays Court to help us find some place to live. We had talked about getting a rancher that was handicap accessible or a mobile home and make it handicap accessible.

He said his dad lived a long life after he moved down south and felt the warmer climate would do him good too. We dreamed of a home with a porch. I could just sit and watch the grass grow and he would shoot at the squirrels. Judy and David told us they would gladly assist us with a search for a home when we were ready.

In the meantime, we discussed the need to make my home handicap accessible. I told him I had an office and he could have that for his work area and counseling sessions.

Since at KHCC, he had gained recognition as a preacher, some called him a priest. He often prayed with residents, their families, and staff. He was even asked to teach at their Wednesday afternoon Bible Study.

He also counseled countless people. Those who came to him knew he could be trusted and asked for prayer. His down to earth manner made people feel comfortable sharing their troubles.

On one of our cafeteria dates, we met a Kennedy employee as she was walking towards the parking lot. We smiled and spoke. Ernest being Ernest and being led by the Holy Spirit initiated a conversation.

She shared that her mother had been a resident at KHCC and had recently passed away. He asked permission to pray for her. We held hands and prayed outside in the courtyard. He also gave her a copy of the *Daily Bread*. He rarely left "home" without some.

About a month later, Ernest was admitted to Kennedy and who do you think was the technician who did his EKG? I was at work but he couldn't wait to tell me the great reunion they had. She told him that when she arrived home after that prayer her husband said, "What happened to you? You have such a glow about you."

She told him of the encounter in the parking lot and showed him the *Daily Bread*. She stated that they have been reading it together either before work or when they came home in the evening.

This was just one of countless ways God used Ernest to minister. Sharing Christ was as natural as breathing. So he liked the idea of having a place to write and counsel. I also told him I knew how much of him he had lost when he had to give up his apartment. I told him he could pick out another room in the house that he wanted to decorate to his liking.

My daughter Leona took pictures of my home and brought them in for Ernest to see. He chose the living room and he started planning the color scheme. Ernest wanted a blue and white living room and we planned to start looking for furniture as soon as he came home.

We now called it our house, our home. I gave him a set of keys to confirm that it was now our home. Lord willing, I plan to make his dreams of a blue and white living room come true this year.

Joe, his roommate, passed away and Ernest was moved to another room. They decided to make his old room into a female room. His new roommate was a quiet man in his 80s who, with help, got out of bed at 7:30 a.m. and sat in his wheelchair until bedtime.

They became buddies. He and Ernest enjoyed quiet times, chats and prayers together. His roommate being in his 80's referred to Ernest as the "young man" and me as the "young lady." They got along well.

When We Get Married

Things were pretty stable, so we were now back to getting married. We gave the lawyer his fees to file for a divorce. Ernest had been separated for over 10 years. There were no minor children or property.

After hiring the lawyer, we ordered our rings, Silver bands with crosses. The crosses were to be a testimony of our Christian belief. We loved them. When he gave me my engagement ring, which also had the crosses on it, he said, "I'm jealous. I want a ring to wear to show the world I'm engaged." *Spoiled brat!*

I bought him a laptop and said, "Now tell them that you are engaged." He always wanted one and he was excited when he got it. Bro. O'Neal was kind enough to download the info from his desktop to the laptop, so he was a real happy camper. I would bring the lap top to KHCC on the weekends for him to enjoy.

Rena celebrated our engagement with us. Her card "together," sits on my dresser today. You got it, right next to the keepsake box that Klisa gave me. Serena sent us a beautiful letter expressing her happiness for us. We were truly blessed.

Prosthesis/Lawyer

Ernest was admitted on the 18th of December. We spent Christmas and another New Year in the hospital. His left knee had gotten infected and he required aggressive IV antibiotics. He had gone to church a few times and to the movies and the prosthesis had irritated his left knee.

The lawyer informed us the previous paper work was out dated and brought new paper work. We were disappointed because we thought by now we would be picking a wedding date. "In God's time", we agreed.

In January Ernest was told he needed cataract surgery. The left eye was worse than right. He decided to wait. He wanted laser but the VA did not offer that option so Ernest said he would follow up in six months.

In March, Ernest got his smile back. He finally got fitted for his bottom dentures. He told me that someone once told him that he needed to get some bottom teeth that no woman would give him the time of day with a raggedy mouth. I told him some people look beyond the physical and they look at the heart.

"Nobody Knows"

Ernest pressed his way to church on April 8, 2012. Little did we know that would be his last time attending service. We agreed it would be better for him to go without his prosthesis. It just wasn't worth the risk of his knees breaking down again.

I came over to KHCC to help him get dressed. He was a little down and he said, "Do you know how hard it is for a man to put on his pants without legs?" My heart broke with him. Another loss in his life not being able to stand up again.

He enjoyed the service and seeing everyone again and of course just getting out. But nobody, but God, Ernest and I had a clue of what he went through to get there. He would often be sitting in his wheelchair for over an hour waiting for transportation, anxious about if his "bowels would break loose." That always was our prayer, "Lord, hold back the diarrhea." We would request medication for the diarrhea and pain.

When he went out, it was usually with pain in his neck; he had several ruptured cervical discs, back and phantom leg usually accompanied him even at rest. Of course, the wait for transportation to take him back also proved to be a taxing occurrence.

Ernest was so exhausted when he returned. He often wouldn't even eat, which was bad because he never ate or drank before going out because of his fear of diarrhea. He would just sleep. It was often days before he recovered. It took so much out of him.

That day when he went to the ER and spent the night, was one of the worse days for him . From there he went to dialysis.

Great Love

Ernest made a bold move. Since his surgery in August 2010, he had never gone out alone. When he felt good, we would take walks on the Nursing Home grounds, venture down the road to Walgreen's and go in and browse around, go to the movies, the malls, and have a cafeteria date across the street at the hospital. But, he never went out alone.

He often asked me about the buses that ran in front of the hospital. They ran very frequently and they were handicap accessible and, unlike Access Link, you didn't have to schedule a day ahead. That's the way he traveled before his surgery.

Well on May 12th he, against medical advice, left KHCC, took the bus and went to the mall by himself. He often said even when people were telling him things for his own good, "Nobody controls me."

He went to buy me a Mother's day present. I still fill up with tears over what he did just for me. He brought me a beautiful green (my favorite color) sleeveless, (he liked looking at my arms), dress with a bolero jacket. When I came over after work, we talked, had dinner, cuddled together and when I was getting ready to leave he said, "Get that bag out of the closet for me."

I opened the door. No balloons this time, but there was a beautiful gift bag. He said, "That's for you." Again, I was speechless. He said, "Happy Mother's Day!"

When I looked inside, I found the dress. I was over whelmed. He said proudly, "I went to the mall and got it myself." Usually he asked Leona to pick up gifts for me or he would use his credit card and order something or just give me money and tell me to pick out something, He said he wanted to go this time and pick out something himself. Oh, how the tears flowed.

I wore it Sunday to church. When I went over after church he said, "Whoa, girl, you really filled out that top."

It was tight across the top, I said, "Maybe I need to get a breast reduction."

He said, "No, don't do that!" He had told me in the past "the only thing I want to change about you is your name."

Like I told Stephanie and some others, "He's good to me and good for me."

He had planned to come to church and I found his check for that date already made out in his Bible and on New Year's Eve put it in the offering plate. He was so exhausted from his trip to the mall that he decided it best to just rest.

On two occasions we attended the church services at KHCC, visiting churches came every Sunday at 2:00pm with a complete service. Their doctrine was sound and the hymns we sang added to the hour-long service. They acknowledged him as being a preacher in the congregation.

Still Waiting

In June, the lawyer called and promised just one more piece of paper work and that he would hand deliver to the court and we would be on our way.

Ernest and I were getting more and more frustrated with this lawyer. He said, "He knows I'm sick in a nursing home, and Brenda is not contesting the divorce. What's the holdup?"

In July Ernest called his office very upset and spoke to the lawyer's daughter who also worked for him. She admitted the whole process was taking too long. We felt we were stuck. We had already paid him in full and didn't think it fair that we retain another attorney and start the process all over again. We learned the hard way; never pay a lawyer in full before you get what you want. Ernest called the Ethics Committee to report his conduct with our case.

On July 24th I noticed his 3rd left finger was swollen, warm to the touch, and it had a slight odor and I brought it to the nurse's attention. When she checked his vital signs, he had a low-grade fever. He said he would have them look at it in dialysis in the morning. They called me at work and told me he was going to the ER after his treatment and he wanted to go to Washington Township. Stratford was much closer, but since it wasn't a real emergency they respected his wishes.

Again, I was grateful because I could just run over and check on him. When I ran over to check on him who was his doctor, no one but the one who told him on New Year's Eve there was nothing else that could be done for him. Ernest and I laughed. I guess God showed him.

He was admitted and that finger because of the infection had to be removed. They tried to treat the infection with dressings and antibiotics but it could not be saved. They had to amputate to avoid it spreading to other fingers. Another loss. He being a brave soldier joked about it. I often gave him manicures as well as shaved and trimmed his hair. I enjoyed doing it and he knew he could depend on me to keep him looking good. He would often say, "Trim my beard, baby, the way you want it."

When he lost his finger he said, "Just one less finger you have to do. I should get a discount." To the nurses he would stick out his left hand and say, "May the force be with you." To make others feel at ease about his amputations when they pulled back the covers for the first time, he would pick up his legs and say, "Meet stumpy and dumpy." I believe he nicknamed his lost finger "lummy".

We both were grateful that they got all of the infection. His incision healed beautifully, and he still had his ring finger! He was left-handed so his movements were a little more challenging; you'd be surprised how the loss of one finger can make you more compromised. After that lengthy hospitalization, he returned to KHCC with bedsores. Horrific in nature. When he was admitted, he had none, but He left with stage 2 and stage 4. Outraged, I made a formal complaint to the hospital and HealthCare Quality Strategies.

On September 7th we finally got the letter we had been waiting for since October of the previous year, Ernest's divorce had been granted on the 28th of August. We could now set a date and get married.

Back to the ER September 14th, this time we went to Stratford, with chest pain, nausea and vomiting. All his tests were negative so we returned to KHCC the next day.

On September 18th, we went to Monroe Township to apply for our marriage license. Ernest was so weak but he insisted we had waited so long, too long.

In anticipation of marriage I had started the process of making our home handicap accessible. In May, I had carpets removed and replaced with laminate flooring to make it easier for his mobility in his motorized wheel chair. Also I had the doors widened to 36 inches handicap requirements and I obtained permits for the ramp. We chose a modular one, in case we did decide to relocate it could be easily taken down and taken with us. The same company that had the modular ramp offered us the best offer we had found for an adjustable bed. Ernest would need that for comfort, one with which he could raise the head and foot, and last but not least a large screen TV placed on the wall for his enjoyment. We were so happy. The house was ready and so were we.

I wanted a church wedding. When Lee, my first husband, and I married it was by a justice of the peace. Both our families were so into our wedding. We just decided to get married without their drama. At this time Ernest was still weak so we decided to just get married at the nursing home. We were so excited.

We planned to keep it small, immediate family, prayer warriors, those who were on our side from the very beginning. The guest list also included a few others in the church who were happy for us from day one.

A few of the residents and we would each invite two people. Well the word got out. Maybe he and I in our excitement told some others, but more came than we expected came. I found my dress with his favorite color blue the weekend before, from David's Bridal. Thank God for Robin Bullock's suggestion. It was marked down 50%, and when I took it to the cash register it was marked down another 50%.

He decided to wear a suit he had at the house. Rena came over and did my makeup and loaned me a beautiful necklace that was my something borrowed. My shoes were old and my unmentionables new. My daughter, daughter-in-love, and granddaughter were my bride's maids. Latoya, my granddaughter, bought our flowers. Ernest's best men were my son, who also gave me away, and Marcus, Ernest's oldest son.

We were married on a Tuesday. Sherrill reminded us that the Jews preferred to be married on Tuesday. This was the day Jesus turned water into wine at the marriage he attended, *John 2:1*.

Mary Rose, the activities coordinator at KHCC and her staff helped us decorate and set up for the reception that followed. The food was catered by Shop Rite. We ordered a sandwich tray, a wrap tray, a cheese and cracker tray, and a fruit tray. We served bottle water, bottled juices and sodas. My daughter-in-love had a cake made with the inscription "And the two shall be one". Rev. Hargrove officiated.

After all that we had been through, we decided I would march in on "We Have Come This Far By Faith" and that we would recess on "Just Want to Praise Him". The ceremony was beautiful and we were prepared to say our own vows but didn't. That was OK, because we were finally married.

At the reception, Ernest leaned over and said, "Do you think Mary Rose could get us a room in the Rehab Unit for the night?" Their rooms were much nicer than the ones at the nursing home.

I said, "I don't know, that might be really pushing it."

We got married at 4 and by 6 Ernest was starting to get tired, so we headed back to his room so he could get undressed and get back in bed. When we were getting him undressed, we saw that he was bleeding from his left perm cath site, so to the ER we had to go. Rena was the only one we told. She took the wedding gifts home and brought back my car, and I met Ernest at the ER still in my wedding dress.

Ernest told the ER staff, "Look, we just got married a few hours ago," proudly showing off his ring and holding my hand up to show off mine. We were only there for a few hours. The doctor put a stitch at the catheter site. We laughed and said we could tell the story to our great-grand's of how we spent our wedding night in the ER. We weren't about to allow anything to "rain on our parade". We were finally married.

We both agreed getting married at KHCC blessed more people than if we had gotten married at the church. After all that the staff and residents had seen us go through, it made their hearts genuinely happy to see us get married.

I had brought in our dinner earlier and left it in the patient refrigerator, so when we did return to KHCC we ate our first dinner together as husband and wife.

Ernest kept asking me, "Are you happy baby?"

I answered, "Yes."

I asked him, "Are you happy?"

He said, "Yes, as long as you are."

I stayed until 4 a.m. He had dialysis. I, the blushing bride, got to go home and sleep in. I was off from work!

Rev. Ernest W. Lewis I and Ms. Lydia Howard
Wedding Ceremony of LOVE
October 2, 2012
4:00pm

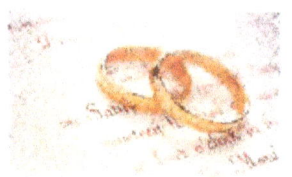

Procession of bridal party:
Best Man – Marcus Lewis
Bride's Maid - Leona Brown
Groom's Man - Leon Howard
Bride's Maid - Cheryl Howard
Ring bearer - Kenny Wayne Faulkner
Flower Girl – La'Ahni Morton

Procession of the Bride
(We Come This Far By Faith)
Prayer -
Scripture -
Solo -
Vows -

Presentation of Bride and Groom
(Just want to Praise You)

Officiating:
Rev. Dr. Robert F. Hargrove, Sr.
Christ Care Unit Missionary Baptist Church

You're Missing God in All of This

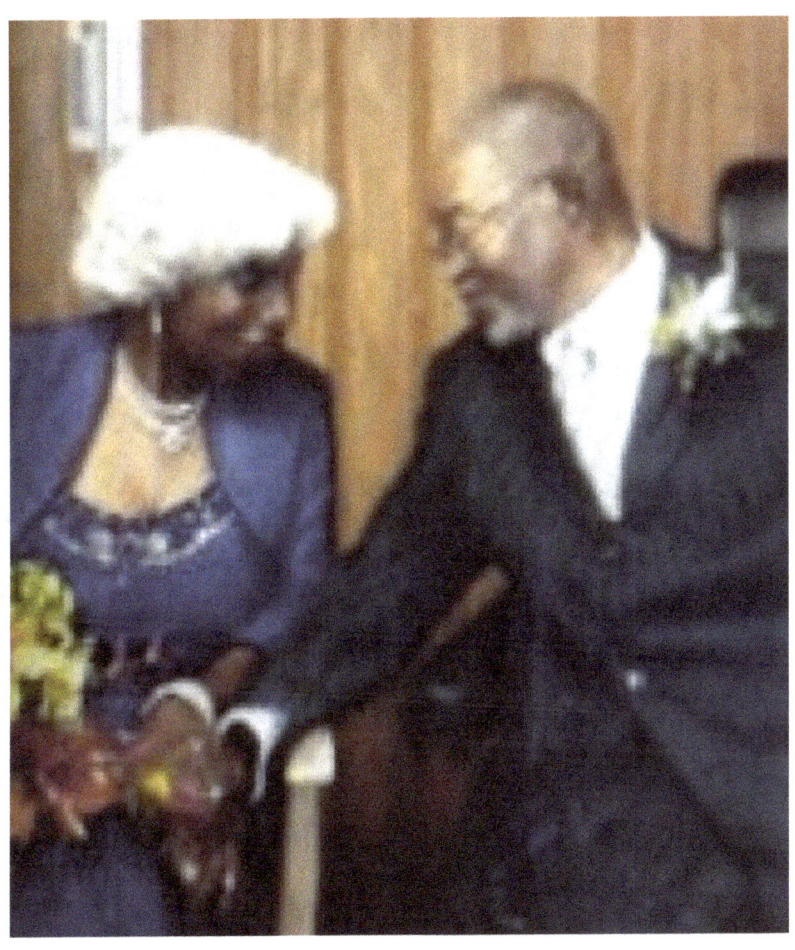

Lydia M. Lewis

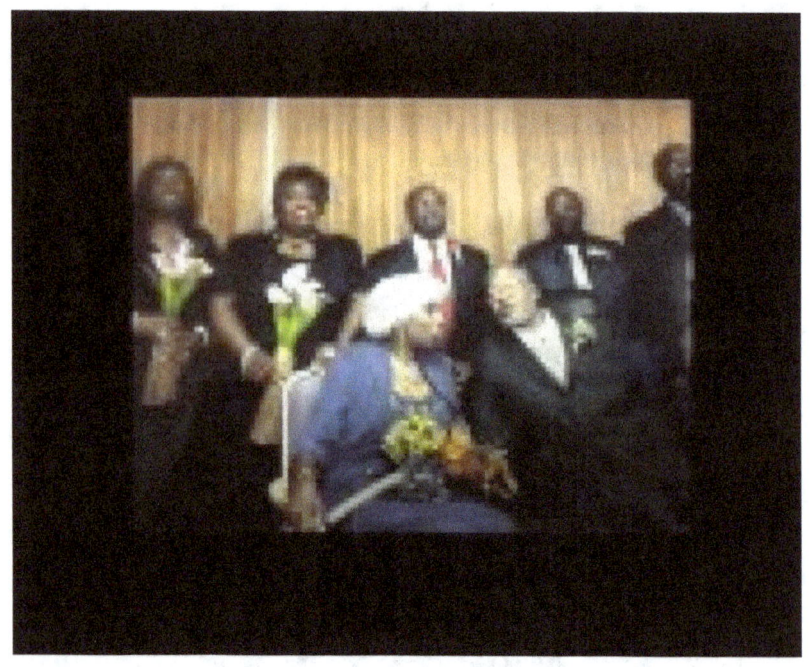

"Lord, Please Give Ernie a Break"

On October 5th, there were problems with the perm cath again. Ernest had to go to Interventional Radiology to get it replaced. The stitch did not hold, it was leaking.

On October 15th back to the ER with chest pain, fluid in his right lung, and a chest tube had to be placed. The nurse practitioner who took care of Ernest and who I also had known and worked with since starting at Kennedy, took me to the side at work one day and said " Ernie's been through so much, I've been asking "Lord please give him a break" She told Ernest, "get out of that nursing home and go home!" And that's what we started working on. The house was already, we were married and we both wanted that more than anything. We talked to the social worker and she started the paper work.

On October 29th, Hurricane Sandy foiled our plans. Ernest was going to come home for the day, but an act of God said no.

That week I had some major car problems, and I had to replace a battery, buy new tires, the left wheel was bent and the car was leaking gasoline. Ernest said, "You know what you have to do. Get a new car and don't buy another green one."

So, on the 3rd of November, I became the owner of a black 2013 Suzuki SX4. Ernest loved it. Before I signed on the dotted line, I called him and told him what they were offering, Leon and Leona went with me. Ernest approved my choice and away I drove off from the dealership. I showed him the brochure and he was pleased. He said, "You did good, it's not green!"

On November 4th to the ER, build up of fluid in the lungs again. Recognizing this would be a chronic problem, a pleurcath was placed. It would have to be drained every other day to every three days to prevent the build up of fluid in his lungs. When he came home I would learn how to do this. I assured him we will get through this! He was now oxygen dependent. During this admission his dialysis catheter also had to be removed and a new one placed because it had gotten infected.

On November 20th, the nurse practitioner wrote the script for the Hoyer lift needed to get Ernest in and out of bed. We still were trying so hard to get him home. The social worker from Medicare had come to finalize the paper work, but we missed her because Ernest was in the hospital.

Home for Thanksgiving

Ernest was coming home for Thanksgiving! We both were so excited. Finally, after 23 months, he was coming home!

I worked Thanksgiving eve, but worked furiously to get off early. KHCC helped him get packed, which basically meant diapers and his meds. He had plenty of clothes at the house.

He arrived about 5:30 p.m. His ride, even though scheduled for 4 p.m., was late. He arrived cold and in pain. Once he got in and took a tour, he felt better.

Ernest loved the house, especially the office. I cleared two walls for him to place his certificates and pictures on. He liked how open it was, with plenty of room for him to get around in his wheelchair. Leona, Leon, and Darnell had removed the hutch in the kitchen, making it more spacious.

He couldn't wait to get into the adjustable bed and watch the big screen TV that was on the wall. He was tired. Thank God my son Leon had stopped over, because

I found out then how weak he was when I tried to help him get in bed.

 Leon picked him up and put him in bed. I got him undressed and he was able to stretch out and relax. Yes, we definitely need a Hoyer lift. He dosed off and when he awoke in a few hours, I gave him his medicine. He was too tired to eat, so we just snuggled and went to sleep. Finally, we got to snuggle together in a real bed.

 In the morning, I made his favorite breakfast. It consisted of grits and two eggs, over easy. I arranged my work schedule so that I would be off at least one of his dialysis days so we could have breakfast together. More importantly, I knew exactly what he liked. When he returned from dialysis, he was often tired and hungry.

 He had stopped eating a lot of meat. He blamed me for that, saying, "You're turning me into a veggie."

 I helped him get bathed and dressed. He helped me set up the indoor turkey fryer I had just purchased the week before. Thank you, Rudy, for suggesting the indoor turkey fryer. While I scrambled around the kitchen to prepare dinner, he watched his big screen TV. Thank God for Cheryl, Leona and later Latoya they came by a little early to help with dinner.

 Ernest had seen a recipe on TV for stuffing, so I bought the ingredients. He sat in the kitchen and directed me. This was the first time I had dinner at our house.

Ernest led us into a Thanksgiving circle prayer and sat at the head of the table. He didn't eat for fear of diarrhea. He would eat later when back at KHCC.

We had a grand time. Rev and Sheila Washington joined us for dinner; our children were there with their families. He watched the girls, Leona, Cheryl, Latoya, practice dancing for Cheryl's big 50th birthday party the following week.

Good food, Good fellowship, Good times.

Access link was two hours late picking Ernest up to return to KHCC. He was slipping out of his seat when placed in the van and they got lost transporting him back. When he finally arrived, his chair didn't work and it took four people to pick him up and get him back in bed. So, needless to say, he was annoyed and tired. He just wanted to go to sleep.

After he got comfortable, I left. I had to go to work and he was scheduled for dialysis. Again, we were determined not to let the devil get the victory. He finally came home and for that we were thankful. He did enjoy it. Finally! After being in one hospital to another, one rehab to another and then the nursing home from September 2010 to November 2012, he made it home.

God didn't have to do that but HE did and for that we were so grateful!

One More Time

Back to the ER November 27th. Ernest had low oxygen levels, and he was lethargic, with a blood sugar down to 33. He was dehydrated, so he was admitted.

God truly saved the best for last. The nursing staff on the 4th floor was the best he had ever had in the two years he had been back and forth as a patient at Kennedy Washington Township. They truly personified the 4 Cs: Caring, Compassion, Commitment and Communication. We were blessed. He was well taken care of on each shift.

On the 1st of December, he made an unusual request. He asked me to go to his room at KHCC and get the "stuff" to make a batch of his cream. This was very unusual, because he didn't like me going to KHCC when he was admitted to the hospital because he knew that "they" would be trying to get information about his condition.

He had instructed me when he first got admitted who to give information to. That was Pastor Hargrove and Ernest's immediate family. He said, "If anybody else wants to know, let them call me or come visit."

So, when people asked, I would simply say, "He's coming along."

The other thing that made this request unusual was that he never made the cream, "Balm N Gilead" while he was in the hospital. We always made it when he was in his room at Manor Care or KHCC. However, I went to KHCC after work the next day and got the "stuff".

When Ernest was at Manor Care, he asked me to buy some African Shea Butter from the beauty supply store, as well as a few other oils and lotions to make his own cream. His skin was so dry and said he would make his own remedy.

It worked. It did wonders for his skin. When he saw how it improved his skin, he shared it with staff. When they came to bathe him, they used his cream instead of the lotion their facility supplied.

He then branched out and started making batches. I would shop around for small containers and he would use them as samples to distribute to staff at Manor Care, dialysis, and KHCC. Those who testified to its success offered to buy it.

I then started shopping for containers of various sizes: sample, small, medium, and large. We once took a trip to the container store in Deptford for containers. We were also blessed to find colorful containers in some local dollar stores.

He prayed over it and named the cream "Balm N Gilead". He was so excited whenever he made a sale! One of the ambulance drivers tried it and wanted to partner with him. She made Shea Butter soap. She also got him a fantastic deal on Shea Butter by the bulk, straight from the motherland, Africa.

One of the staff at Manor care who tried and liked it also wanted to partner with Ernest. His sister owned a beauty salon and was sure there would be a market for it in her salon.

Ernest enjoyed so much making it. It was tedious because he made it by hand. It took hours to mix the other ingredients smoothly in with the Shea Butter, but he didn't mind. When he got tired of stirring and mixing, I would take over. It did my heart good to see him take such an interest in his venture.

The day I bought the "stuff" over, he was tired. When I spread the ingredients out, we had just enough for another batch — a quart. He said, "I'm too weak, you're going to have to make it. I want to give Debbie (his most loyal customer) and Leona some and I'm not going to sell it anymore. I'm just going to give it away."

I told him, "That is fine and I will make it."

Debbie and Leona both had been asking for more, because their supply had run out. So, I mixed it and he was glad we had just enough to make one batch. I mixed and mixed that Saturday night until I got tired and I told him I would finish mixing until it got smooth.

The next day, Sunday December 2nd, I arrived after church and I found him lethargic. The nurse reported that he was not eating and that she had to give him orange juice for his low blood sugar. I knew he hadn't eaten dinner the day before and I had brought him dinner that day. He just ate a few mouthfuls and kept dosing off.

The next day, I tried to reach him from work by phone and kept getting his voicemail. I thought, *He's probably in dialysis I'll wait for his call.* He never called.

When I went over after work, I found out that in dialysis they were unable to remove any fluid because his blood pressure was in the 70s, he wasn't eating and he became nauseated and was vomiting. The doctor ordered blood work.

I was able to get him to at least eat a protein gelatin and then he said barely above a whisper, "You're determined to get me healthy aren't you?"

I responded by saying, "I most certainly am." He just dosed back off to sleep.

The next day he called me at work and said he slept well and had eaten breakfast, a bowl of Farina. This was not his favorite, which was oatmeal, but he knew he had to get something in his stomach. I applauded him for that. I told him I would write out the check for KHCC from his account and take it over after work.

From the beginning, Ernest or I wrote out the checks for KHCC, even though they were taking every cent, except $35. He still wanted that control. When I took the check over, I went to see the social worker. Ernest had been begging since this admission to go home. He would say, "I want to go home, not my heavenly home, but our home." He said, "I don't want to die in the hospital or KHCC, but at home. Is that ok with you?"

I said, "That is perfectly fine with me, no problem."

He thought his time was getting close. He had thought about it many times before in the past 2 years, but this time he shared with me this reoccurring dream. He told me on two different occasions that he had a dream that he was walking again. He said, "I don't know if this is the way the Lord is preparing me to go to heaven or maybe I'll be getting some new legs."

He had said so many times before if some new prosthesis "comes out that will not cause my knees to break down and get infected, I will gladly be the guinea pig." I just held his hand and rubbed his head as he liked me to do. I couldn't respond, because as much as I would have liked to deny it, he was getting so much worse.

When I shared his wish to go home with the social worker, she stated he would first have to return to KHCC. As soon as he did, she would initiate the process again immediately.

I shared my conversation with the social worker with Ernest, but he was not satisfied. He said, "I'm going to just sign myself out."

I said, "Babe, we don't have the support you need to be comfortable and safe because we need the social worker to get everything set up first." He sulked and ate a half of an egg salad sandwich without bread and drank a glass of iced tea, for which I was so grateful, because he was eating again.

Infectious disease came in and informed Ernest of a new medication for his chronic diarrhea. Ernest and I were excited about it. He was scheduled to get his first dose tomorrow before dialysis.

The next day, I called Ernest from work. He sounded groggy, but said he had eaten a bowl of oatmeal for breakfast and was now getting the new medication via IV before getting his dialysis treatment.

When I arrived at the hospital after work, he was lethargic, had labored breathing with his nasal O_2 and was not looking good. Not looking good at all. I was trying so hard not to panic, but I knew I had to call his family.

First I called Brenda, next Lucy, then his sons and Aunt Honey, and lastly, Pastor Hargrove for prayer. I can't remember if I called Leona or if she called me. In any event, she came right over.

I learned from the dialysis nurse that he didn't have much of a treatment. His blood pressure was low and he refused to stay on the machine. His blood pressure indeed was low when I arrived and the doctor was called. He wanted Ernest transferred to the intensive care unit.

Leona came and Ernest told me to give her the cream. I had a jar prepared for her. Leona, seeing how sick he was, said, "Now you know you have to get stronger so you can make some more of this cream." He smiled.

Leona and I chatted when he appeared to drift off to sleep and then he awoke and said, "Talk about something spiritual." We did and Leona even sang a song. Rev. Washington called to check on Ernest as he so often did and when he talked with me he said he would be right over. He came and prayed a prayer that brought calm and a peace over us all: Ernest, Leona, and myself.

Ernest was transferred to the intensive care unit with one unsuccessful attempt after another to place an IV access. They couldn't even place one under ultrasound. Ernest was very quiet throughout the whole ordeal. The doctors said, "You're a real trooper."

When they finally gave up, he looked at me and said, "Lydia I'm getting worse."

Fighting back the tears I said, "Sometimes you have to get worse before you get better."

He firmly repeated, "Lydia I'm getting worse." I just continued to rub his head and hold his right hand as I always did when he was in pain or upset.

Aunt Honey called back with her cell phone number, and Brenda called back saying they were making plans to "pull out the next morning." About 11 p.m., I thanked Leona for coming and staying with me but told her that she should go. It was going to be a long night.

I had called my nurse manager before he even got transferred to the ICU when I saw how poorly Ernest was and told her I wouldn't be in for work as scheduled the next day. She understood and offered her support. My second call out in 11 years. The first one was when my first husband, Leon, was in the ER and was being admitted.

I was hopeful. Even the staff was encouraged when Ernest's blood pressure came up to the 80s and 90s without intervention. He still had no IV access.

They needed labs so they called the dialysis nurse on call and she came in to draw labs. She was the nurse manager. We had worked together. She not only drew the labs, but also offered her support and said, "If you need anything do not hesitate to call."

A chest x-ray was conducted and it showed no significant changes. They planned to send Ernest to radiology for a line placement when they opened in the morning.

Marcus called and I urged him to come ASAP. Things were not looking good. Ernest was basically quiet, dozing off. When he awoke, he saw that I was still there. I just continued to hold his hand and rub his head. We had told each other so many times how much we loved one another, and how we had been blessed in the short time we had together with more happiness than other couples who had been together so much longer and enjoyed better health and so many less hospital admissions. So, we really didn't do a lot of talking, just receiving the time God was still allowing us to hold on to each other.

Ernest was now barely responsive and the doctors asked permission to use his dialysis access to draw labs. I agreed, desperate to do whatever it took to keep him alive. As I was holding his hand, he pulled away. My mother did the same thing as I held her hand the last few minutes of her life on earth. It was if they both were telling me the same thing, "Let me go. I'm on my way home."

The dialysis nurse came about 7:45 a.m. to give him a more gentle dialysis CVVHD. After he had set up the machine and before starting treatment, Ernest's blood pressure dropped down to 61. As the medical staff all ran in, I was moved to the foot of the bed and he mouthed something. If I would dare to speculate what it was, it would be what he said so many times when he was at his lowest point, "Lord I hope I've done enough."

As I went to approach him, they called a code and I stepped out of the room and watched. They confirmed, "His wishes were not to be intubated?"

I said, "Yes. Those were his wishes." They did everything they could.

He was pronounced dead at 8:23 a.m.

The End?

> *"To everything there is a season,*
> *and a time to every purpose under the heaven;*
> *A time to be born. And a time to die."*
> — Ecclesiastes: 3: 1-2
>
> *Precious in the sight of the Lord*
> *is the death of His faithful saints.*
> — Psalms 116:15

I wept softly. The staff doctors and nurses offered their support. So many of them had known Ernest for years and knew he fought a good fight and had now finished his course.

Ernest had instructed me not to grieve in public. He said "I know you can be strong I saw you bury your husband and daughter, do your grieving privately at home."

In our many conversations months before, Ernest stated that he wanted three things, for us to get married, to make it home, our home and to die at home. I pray that his wanting to die at home was because he wanted me there. I was there! I agree with Dave Brannon, who said, "When death comes for a follower of Christ, God opens His arms to welcome that person into His presence."

As I cried out to the Lord in the days and weeks after, "All we wanted was to be together!" We weren't asking for a luxurious home, a big bank account, or even to be able to travel. We just wanted to be together, wake up to each other and spend the day having our Bible study, watching TV, eating our favorite foods together, and just talking.

God answered, "I gave you precious time and precious love together. So many people saw your love for one another and were encouraged as Jasmine once said, 'To actually see pure and true love.'"

In the words of Maya Angelo, "I wouldn't take nothing for the journey."

I believe with all my heart that now my greatest desire for Ernest has been fulfilled and that was that he "be happy and comfortable." Ernest and I did not *"miss God in all of this."* I pray in your story that you may want to share one day that you don't *"miss God in all of this."*

I am so blessed!

I have been not only left with a lifetime of beautiful memories but also with a new and loving family. Madea, Ernest's mom in Georgia; Aunt Honey, his dad's sister;

Ernest's sisters, Brenda, Lucy, Patsy, Shirley, and Bernice; a brother, Claude; his best friend of over 40 years, Sherrill; his sons, Marcus and Ernie; and a host of grandchildren, great-grands, nephews and nieces.

On 10 January 2007 at 6:38 a.m., Ernest wrote and left this note among his papers, "The pastor who does my funeral preach this 'A Place Prepared for Me' John 14:1- 4." That was the Eulogy Rev. Dr. Robert F. Hargrove Sr. preached on 10 December 2012.

Dedication

This book is dedicated to our Lord and Savior, Jesus Christ.

"For in Him we live, and move, and have our being ... for we are also His offspring."
— Acts 17:28

It was *Him* who gave Ernest and I precious love and precious time.

God is everywhere. Wherever you are, GOD is! He loves you and has demonstrated that love in a way no one else has by dying on the cross for your sins. He is faithful and continues to care, protect and provide for you. When He arose from the grave, He proved that He truly does have all power in His hands. Ernest and I did not miss God in this short time he gave us together. How could we? **He** was there with us through it **all.** My prayer is that you not miss God. He's there. Stop, Look, and Listen as you travel along your life's journey.

There is no cost for this book.
As our first lady, Sis. Hargrove, so frequently reminds us, as God so freely gives to us, this book is freely given to you.

"Freely ye have received, freely give."
— Matthew 10:8

If book has allowed you to "See God in all of This," please consider making a donation to the **Kennedy Dialysis Center's Patient Assistance Fund.** Donations made in memory of Rev. Ernest Wayne Lewis 1st will be deeply appreciated. Your tax-deductible contribution will be able to assist patients with emergency short term transportation, medications costs, and crisis relief.

For further information please contact **Jeffrey Jin**, social worker at **(856) 566-5467** or mail your donation to:

Voorhees Dialysis Center
201 Laurel Oak Rd
Voorhees NJ 08043

In memory of Rev. Ernest W. Lewis 1st

www.ingramcontent.com/pod-product-compliance
Lightning Source LLC
Chambersburg PA
CBHW052056070526
44584CB00017B/2203